BODY
TRANSFORMATIONS

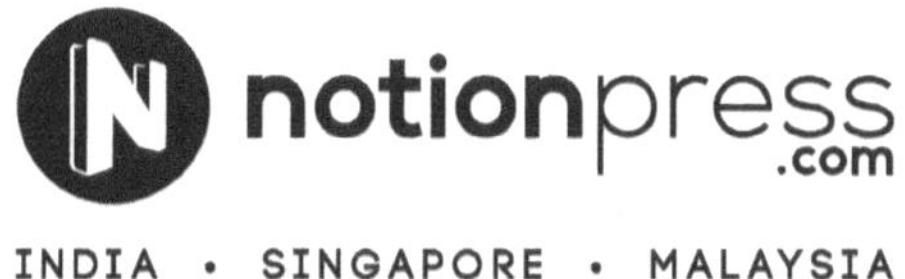

INDIA • SINGAPORE • MALAYSIA

Notion Press

No.8, 3rd Cross Street,
CIT Colony, Mylapore,
Chennai, Tamil Nadu – 600004

First Published by Notion Press 2020
Copyright © Vishal Gupta 2020
All Rights Reserved.

ISBN 978-1-64951-708-1

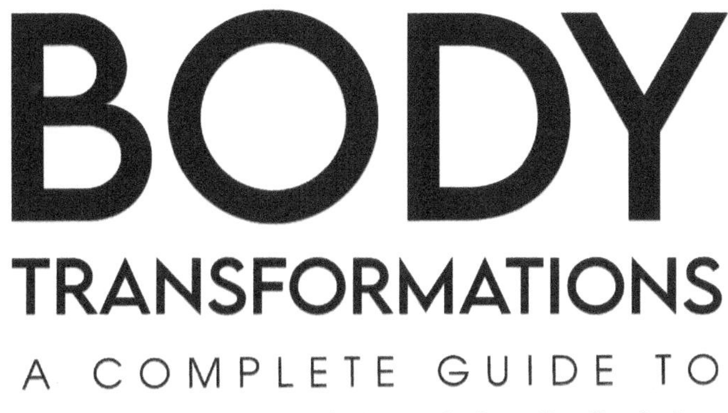

BODY TRANSFORMATIONS

A COMPLETE GUIDE TO YOUR FITNESS GOAL

VISHAL GUPTA

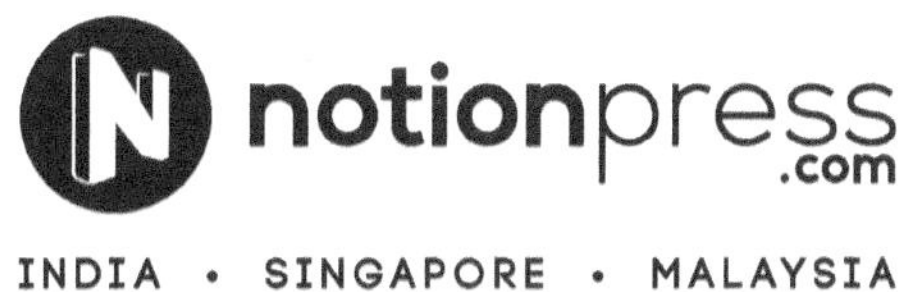

INDIA · SINGAPORE · MALAYSIA

INDICACADEMY

Indic Pledge

- *I celebrate our civilisational identity, continuity & legacy in thought, word and deed.*

- *I believe our indigenous thought has solutions for the global challenges of health, happiness, peace and sustainability.*

- *I shall seek to preserve, protect and promote this heritage and in doing so,*
  - *discover, nurture and harness my potential,*
  - *connect, cooperate and collaborate with fellow seekers,*
  - *advance diversity and inclusivity in the society.*

About Indic Academy

Indic Academy is a non-traditional 'university' for traditional knowledge. We seek to bring about a global renaissance based on Indic civilizational and indigenous thought. We are pursuing a multidimensional strategy across time, space and cause by establishing centers of excellence, transforming intellectuals and building an ecosystem.

Indic Academy is pleased to support this book.

CONTENTS

AUTHOR'S NOTE

Ever since I gained consciousness, I found myself inclined towards fitness. In my early days, I did not find a coach. One of my peers gifted me a book written by Mr. Arnold Schwarzenegger titled *The encyclopedia of Bodybuilding* and, with this book, he became my idol and, till date, I am a big fan.

I started following all his ideologies from the very beginning and, here I will mention one of his rules, which was giving back to society. This thing was deep inside me, that whatever I have gained in life, Once I will be capable enough, I will return to mankind. Gradually I took many national and, international certifications, and, at the same time performed as a fitness athlete and, finally became a fitness expert with time and, took it professionally too.

My book *Body Transformation: A Complete Guide to Your Fitness Goals* is the journey I have been through and, all the external and, internal parameters I took care of, that turned me from a common man to a fitness expert.

Getting fit is slowly becoming the most challenging task nowadays. Gradually, as the fitness industry is growing, it is also being highly commercialized also. At the same time with the increasing importance of social interaction, everyone wants to look presentable and, fashionable and, to leave an impression on social networking sites.

Each one of us wants to look fit, but are not able to actually get fit, because either it's made really complicated, technical and, expensive or now fitness is not about hard work, dedication and, consistency. It's all about superfoods, supplementation and, fancy work outs. According to me, people do not follow a planned approach, it's only based on hit and, trial methods.

This assessment of mine made me write a book which covers all the aspects of body transformation, through which you can not only look fit and, fabulous, but also maintain the same throughout your all life.

In February 2019, one of my friends with his wife approached me for body transformation. To assess their present position, I started with a new angle, that is blood reports and, it benefitted them and, gave desired results. Yes, when it comes to body transformation we all take care of work out and, meal planning, but no one take cares about internal body systems and, how they affect our goals. How our heart, lungs, kidney, stomach and, other hormones speed up or delay the process.

Writing the book was there in my mind for long, but how I began is really emotional.

In August 2019, one of my best friends, a college mate, was hospitalized. When I spoke to him he told me about the problems. I called him to send his reports. He sent some, and, I gave him a list of blood tests to get done. Meanwhile, to get fit, he got a new cycle, started to work out, but the tests were not done. One day I got a message from his mobile that he is no more. I was shaken badly and, I could not handle myself. I decided this should not happen to anyone else and, I started writing the book.

Obesity never comes alone, with itself, it brings several complications. Eventually, after having put on a sizable amount of fat, our body begins to signal us about the problem. Then, it's time to react, to take action, and, transform into the fitter version of ourselves that is better suited to our body structure. This book is a perfect guide to help you achieve your best looks, no matter what you look like or where you work out.

Happy Health

Regards

Vishal Gupta

ACKNOWLEDGMENTS

I thank my family and, my loved ones always supporting me and, motivating me.

PREFACE

Hello Everyone

On 23-3-2020, Geenika's birthday, I started writing this book

"Body Transformation – A Complete guide to your fitness goals"

In this fast-paced and, competitive world, everyone wants to be appreciated about their looks and, leave long-lasting first impression. Every individual has a wish to look good, whether to attain a short term goal or to just fit into a particular outfit.

Everyone strives to acquire a fast-acting temporary solution to look great, but the fact remains that, being enigmatically fit is the only way to achieve that fascinating personality.

Body Transformation, I consider it as a road trip from Delhi to Ladakh, it's fascinating, adventurous and, beautiful but at the same time really challenging, risk-taking and, full of hurdles too.

Before starting, we need to check our car's or bike's condition, the same way we need to check our body's present parameters like fat %, internal body functioning, endurance, strength and, flexibility. We need to have a schedule for daily distance coverage and, all the possible halts, similarly we need to pursue all the short term and, long term goals with work out designing and, meal planning. All the emergency situations in the trip need to be planned similarly injuries and, disorders need to be dealt with in body transformation. Above all, mind and, motivation matter in both cases.

This book is a complete road map, with all the dos and, don'ts for the trip called Body Transformation.

We assure you, after reading this book, Body Transformation will no more be a nightmare and, you can remain fit and, fabulous forever. Happy Health, Good luck

– **Vishal Gupta**

WHAT IS OBESITY ACTUALLY?

There is a table called Height weight table, that is what should be your weight corresponding to your height, it's for both men and, women.

WOMEN				MEN			
Height Ft. In.	Small	Med.	Large	Height Ft. In.	Small	Med.	Large
4'10"	102-111	109-121	118-131	5'2"	128-134	131-141	138-150
4'11"	103-113	111-123	120-134	5'3"	130-136	133-143	140-153
5'0"	104-115	113-126	122-137	5'4"	132-138	135-145	142-156
5'1"	106-118	115-129	125-140	5'5"	134-140	137-148	144-160
5'2"	108-121	118-132	128-143	5'6"	136-142	139-151	146-164
5'3"	111-124	121-135	131-147	5'7"	138-145	142-154	149-168
5'4"	114-127	124-138	134-151	5'8"	140-148	145-157	152-172
5'5"	117-130	127-141	137-155	5'9"	142-151	156-160	155-176
5'6"	120-133	130-144	140-159	5'10"	144-154	151-163	158-180
5'7"	123-136	133-144	143-163	5'11"	146-157	154-166	161-184
5'8"	126-139	136-150	146-167	6'0"	149-160	157-170	164-188
5'9"	129-142	139-153	149-170	6'1"	152-164	160-174	168-192
5'10"	132-145	142-156	152-173	6'2"	155-168	165-178	172-197
5'11"	135-148	145-159	155-176	6'3"	158-172	167-182	176-202
6'0"	138-151	148-162	158-176	6'4"	162-176	171-187	181-207

Height-Weight-Chart-In-Pounds

When you get your blood test done, all your parameters have a certain reference range similarly after a certain age our height is fixed, according to that height, our bodyweight should fall in certain acceptable or reference range. This is called the height-weight table.

For example, the weight of a male of height 5 feet 10 inches should be between 68 kg to 75kg. These are the minimum and, the maximum values for small and, large frame respectively. Now, both ways it is not good, neither less than 68 nor more than 75.

When your bodyweight exceeds 75 kgs in this case, we term it as overweight or obesity.

If the weight goes above 75, unless we train ourselves to gain muscle weight for a purpose, that means it is not good for us and, body fat is increasing. The first implication is, that our skeletal structure is designed to hold a maximum 75 kg weight, and, if it goes beyond that it puts extra pressure on our skeletal structure, secondly, our internal body parts also have to work more to sustain that increased bodyweight.

It's like doing overtime in your office, to handle the extra work load. Any one can do overtime for 2-3 hours once or twice a week but imagine if you have to do overtime daily that too for 6-8 hours, what will happen. After some time you will not be able to handle.

Same happens with our body, first our skeletal system which is bearing the load of those extra kilos, for which it is not designed, will start to give signals, like body aches, joint pains, weakness etc.

Then our internal body parts like heart, liver, kidney, lungs, intestine, and, the hormonal system will also collapse one by one after a point of time.

This is a bitter truth.

As I said in the start "Overweight or Obesity never comes alone", it increases the risk of many other health problems also.

Gaining a few kilos during the year may not seem like a big deal. But these kilos generally adds up over time.

With time, gradually due to sedentary lifestyle and, unhealthy eating habits, we start gaining weight and, with that we start developing certain discrepancy in our internal body system and, it starts giving signals primarily like, fatigue, body pains, muscle weakness, joint issues, stress, depression, sleep disorders and, certain medical complications also like blood pressure, sugar, thyroid, vitamin and, mineral deficiencies, high bad cholesterol levels, hormonal imbalances, liver and, kidney malfunctioning, stomach issues etc.

Now, what happens, some of us ignore these signals, some have peer recommendations for handling the bad signals, some start some self medications taking suggestions from the internet or media and, very rarest or when the problem increases see a doctor.

The problem doesn't ends here, we start treating the symptoms or the signals which body is giving

Like muscle and, bones issues, we start taking pain killers, for stomach issues different home remedies, for stress, depression, sleep disorders, we start low dose medicines and, many more like this.

What is the problem actually?????????????????????????

Is it the signals or the root cause

We never try to find out the root cause, we just try to stop or reduce the symptoms or the body signals.

What has actually happened?

What happens to the internal body system when bodyweight starts increasing?

Our body is a family, where every member has some predefined role or functions to perform.

From a layman's perspective, if any of the family members gets hurt, all the other members collectively come for the rescue and, perform the injured member's functions.

In this case, a simple conclusion, that the functioning will not be 100%, and, gradually the discrepancy will increase and, overall body functioning will be disturbed, initially to a level and, with time a complete breakdown.

Let's look at these family members which contributes to our basic health,

Heart – controls the blood circulation in the body, with an increase in cholesterol levels, it's functioning reduces

Gastro-Intestinal Tract – The food metabolism engine and, the energy bank, with calorie mismanagement, our stomach issues starts

Thyroid Gland – which controls the body metabolism and, digestive functions, with its malfunctioning the bodyweight gets disturbed, it can be hereditary also

Pancreas which secretes Insulin which controls the amount of sugar or glucose in blood, in cases of disturbance, the body's cells does not accept the glucose causing insulin resistance, signaling sugar issues

Liver, which breakdowns fat and, filters our digestive tract, due to our toxic diet unhealthy lifestyle, its not able to function properly and, leads to various problems.

Kidney, it passes waste from body and, also filter blood before sending it back to heart and, also maintain fluid balance, with time it does not function properly because of overload and, various issues starts leading to medical complications as well.

Adrenal Gland, producing cortisol which manage our metabolism, immune system, blood pressure, response to stress and, other essential functions, with increasing stress levels and, sedentary lifestyle the internal body system gets badly hampered.

Our reproductive hormones, with time and, age if they are not being in sufficient quantity it leads to many problems

Vitamins and, Minerals, the micro nutrients, some produced by the body and, some obtained from diet are mostly ignored, their deficiency also disturb our health

Taking about our subject, all the above parameters play a big role in maintaining our health and, fitness

In most of the cases of obesity, one or more than one of the above parameters are seen to be disturbed.

Everyone want's to look fit, be problem-free and, carry on with the basic daily activities to their best.

Everyone says I want to look fit, but the question is "Do we want to be Fit"

What is the difference?

Yes, there is.

What is the meaning of fitness?

Let's come straight to the point, Body has basically two types of weight, one is fat weight and, the other is muscle weight.

For males – the acceptable fat weight ratio is 10-12%

For Females – the acceptable fat weight ratio is 18-20%

If you maintain this fat weight ratio in your body you are fit.

Also at this acceptable fat weight ratio all the above family members or the body machinery system are working fine.

Now with lifestyle and, eating habits when the fat weight ratio starts increasing above this acceptable range, one or more than one family member starts getting disturbed which gradually takes a giant form.

As this giant is becoming big, time to time body gives signals, that please help.

Here I would mention that in some special cases, it may happen that, when one of the family member or body's machinery part is not working properly due to some hereditary conditions, or some sudden incident or accident or some prolonged medication, the body's fat weight ratio may get disturbed.

Now when we all can see there is problem, the body has started giving SOS signals for help.

Now the most important aspect is, to identify the SOS signals, find out how many family members are not working properly and, start taking actions for the corrective measures regarding lifestyle and, eating habits.

Here I would mention, in 99.99% cases, where the body is giving signals, the most common problem is Obesity or the increasing fat percentage inside the body.

Plan of action for body transformation

Also the mission of looking fit or in my terms "getting Fit" is only achievable through the following plan of action:

CHAPTER 1

IDENTIFY THE BODY FAT PERCENTAGE

Identify the body fat percentage

1. The first and, almost correct way is – Body composition Analysis, A machine which tells us about the body fat weight, weight of the muscles, bones and, tendons, body water, also we get to know the visceral fat – the fat above the organs, which is there to guard the organs at a minimum level, but when increases due to our bad lifestyle it can be dangerous medically. In advance BCA machine we get to know many other parameters also which can help us in our Body Transformation.

2. The Height weight ratio that is your BMI

   This can be calculated as weight /square of height in meters

   Like if your weight is 80 kg and, height is 180 cm or 1.8 meters

   Then 80/1.8x1.8 = 24.69

   BMI is 24.69

   Statistics shows – BMI <18-20 is perfect

   BMI – from 20 to 25 is acceptable

   BMI – from 25 to 30 is overweight

   BMI - above 30 is obese and, needs medical attention

   The only draw back with this system is that in case of a person with more muscle mass, like in bodybuilders and, powerlifters, there BMI will be above 25 but they may not be considered overweight as they have more of good weight that is muscle weight than the bad weight that is fat weight. Here Would recommend to rely on other methods also (like the hip waist ratio can be checked) so that the fat percentage should not be above the acceptable range.

3. The waist-hip ratio

    We calculate Waist / Hip

    If this ratio lies between 0.8 to 0.9 then it's ok

    If this ratio lies between 0.9 to 1 then it is overweight

    If this ratio is above 1 then the person is in the obese category.

4. Skin Fold Test – In this method skin is pinch hold with a Caliper and, than from a pre defined table we can calculate the fat deposition percentage in various parts of the body.

5. Underwater weighing – If a person is weighed underwater, we will only get his muscle mass and, in that case, the fat weight can be calculated.

    By all the above means we can definitely calculate the Body fat % of a person pursuing Body Transformation

How to calculate the target bodyweight

When we have calculated the body fat percentage, now we can asses the correct target weight of an individual. Normally whenever we talk about Body Transformation the terminology is weight loss, nobody says fat loss. When we talk about weight, as mentioned above we have good weight and, bad weight, fat and, muscle weight. Why would someone lose something good?

This actually happens irrespective of the individual physical characteristics we run after a number on the weighing scale.

Universally we have a height weight table for males and, females discussed in first chapter, a layman would certainly try to fit into the weight range that is given in the table, irrespective of his own body type.

Here's an example

For a person with height 5feet10inches, the height-weight table says he should weight between 68 to 75 kg depending on the body frame (lean or bulky)

Now let's assume a male, of same height is 90 kgs, to fit into this table he has to lose atleast 15kgs

Here, comes the importance of body fat percentage analysis. The BCA machine says he has 17 kgs of fat weight, that is 20% fat percentage.

Now, the acceptable male fat % is 10-12% that means, the fat he has to reduce as of now is 8% that is 7.2kg.

As u can clearly see he does not have to lose 15kgs, he just need to lose 7 kgs of fat, I again re insist FAT.

What is the point here to lose 8 kgs extra till he has some specific goal of a lesser fat % like a muscle model or a fitness competition athlete.

Also with this Body fat analysis we get to know our good weight that is muscle weight, In most of the cases, if we do not take care of our diet and, training regime we tend to lose muscles more than fat, which further increases the overall fat % and, we tend to worsen our present condition.

Here I would mention that during our Body Transformation we should check our body fat and, muscle percentage regularly, its really important.

Now when we have defined our goal, how much fat we have to lose, lets focus on our strengths and, weaknesses.

CHAPTER 2

INTERNAL BODY ASSESSMENT

Identifying the body parts or the functions not working properly

When we are heading towards a mission, the most important aspect is to know what are our strong aspects, and, also we need to minimize our weaknesses.

When it comes to body transformation, our internal body system plays an important role. It can be our asset and, it can be our liability too. You must have noticed that some people gets good results with normal efforts and, some people have to put in a lot of effort to get results and, still they do not get what you want.

Let's assume that if some one's thyroid gland is not working properly, in that case the person has to put more effort to manage weight. Also take one case where the problem of insulin resistance is there, here also the problems like blood sugar levels and, insulin spike will make the body transformation journey difficult. That is why it is really important to find out which internal body systems are malfunctioning, then only we will be able to carry on with our journey. If comparing our body transformation to a long drive then how will we be able to carry on longer with leakage of engine oil. So the car should be checked thoroughly before we start and, it should also be checked after regular time intervals, so is our body.

When it comes to Body Transformation, we think our target is to look fit or to lose some weight, this kind of thinking is really temporary.

If we want to transform our body completely and, maintain it throughout life time then it is more important to make sure that our all the internal body parts should function properly and, then only it will be called a successful and, long lasting Body Transformation.

To look Fit you have to get Fit first.

Here the first step is to get the blood tests done for all the body parts as mentioned below –

1. Heart Functioning – Tests – Lipid Profile, which will tell about the cholesterol levels inside the body. Higher bad cholesterol levels (LDL) and, higher Triglyceride levels shows that the body is accumulating fats and, in conjugation, with other tests we can definitely lower them with certain nutrients, diet management and, exercise principles.

    Here an important point is to check the HDL also that is good cholesterol which is beneficial in body transformation. If it's low we need to take care of it also.

2. Gastro-Intestinal Tract – When it comes to Body Transformation, the gastro intestinal tract, from our food pipe to the anus, consist of large intestine and, the small intestine and, other body parts. This is our food metabolism engine and, if there is certain inflammation here or some kind of leakage, then our food will not be metabolized properly which results in fat depositions and, secondly in case of leakage the nutrients like vitamins & minerals are not absorbed properly, which act as key components in functioning of many organs.

    Here we need to check the ESR (erythrocyte sedimentation rate), C-Reactive Protein, Homocysteine.

3. Thyroid Gland -Tests – Thyroid profile and, Thyroid antibodies

The most important gland, when it comes to body transformation and, weight management. It directly affects our goals as the hormones secreted by this gland controls the body metabolism and, digestive functions.

In case of hypothyroidism, when the gland is underactive, what ever we eat is not metabolized properly and, the chances of fat gain increases. Here I would like to mention that in many cases people are taking the thyroid medicines like thyroxin or eltroxin, which is T4, inside the body it is converted to T3 as T3 is 4 times more powerful. Now there are more than 11 key nutrients which execute this transaction, and, if this conversion does not take place effectively, the person is still not able to maintain weight inspite of taking medicine.

There are cases where T3, T4, TSH are within normal range, but in that case we check the thyroid antibodies, it is possible that the antibodies have increased which shows possibilities of auto-immune disease.

If all the above are normal, then Reverse T3 is checked, which shows the clear picture of the gland. In any case this gland plays a really important role and, it's all the parameters should be checked thoroughly.

4. Insulin controls the amount of sugar or glucose in blood and, insulin resistance is a disease when the body's cells does not accept the glucose, in that case the glucose circulates freely in the blood. Brain consider this glucose as unused or not required and, store it in the form of triglycerides and, then fat. In this case the test done are Fasting Insulin, Fasting blood glucose, HBA1C. If these are all above normal values, then nutrients and, diet both need to be altered accordingly. These reports can be studied with the lipid profile for proper diagnosis.

Test to be done – HBA1C, Blood Glucose, Fasting Insulin, Leptin

5. Liver, which breakdowns fat and, filters our digestive tract, need to checked properly. In today's lifestyle, because of all the toxins we intake in many forms the liver malfunctioning is really common. Here we get the Liver functioning Test done, primarily with other factors, we examine the SGPT and, SGOT levels which clearly shows the liver toxicity.

6. Uric acid is a product of the metabolic breakdown of purines and, it's a normal component of urine, but high blood concentrations of uric acid leads to gout, diabetes and, kidney stones. Also it can create disturbance in our work out also because of physical aspects. It needs to be taken care of, properly with other kidney parameters. The test here is a Kidney functioning test.

7. Stress Levels are increasing day by day, in that case the Cortisol levels increase which disturbs our metabolism, immune system, blood pressure and, response to stress.

    In all the above aspects, it is really difficult to continue with our body transformation goals. We need to get our cortisol levels checked and, take the nutrients and, diet accordingly.

8. Our reproductive hormones, if they are not being produced in sufficient quantity it leads to many problems. It may be because of many reasons, our activity level, our lifestyle, our diet, and, are we taking the key nutrients in right proportion. Testestestorone and, Estrogen basically are present in both, males and, females, in males testestorone is more and, in females estrogen is more and, they play their respective characteristics. These need to checked, whether they are in appropriate quantity or not. They play an important role in body transformation.

9. Vitamins and, Minerals, the micro nutrients, some produced by the body and, some obtained from diet are mostly ignored. These micro nutrients are the keys to many metabolic functions which are necessary for optimal health and, body composition. Here, I have talked about thyroid gland, where T4 is converted into T3

inside the body. Here I would say that it takes nearly 11 different minerals and, vitamins like Vitamin A, C, E, zinc, Selenium and, many more, for this effective conversion to take place and, then only the thyroid gland functions properly. Blood circulation, brain sensors, food metabolism, hormone secretion, fat breakage and, many different functions are triggered and, managed by the vitamins and, minerals. In fact they control our total health. If we to get fit for ever these need to be taken care.

10. Food Allergies and, Toxicity: It happens that our body becomes allergic to different foods, which can lead to toxicity and, inflammation inside the stomach. Like many people are lactose intolerant, they are not comfortable having milk. I have seen people allergic to gluten, corn, certain vegatables or fruits, this is really personal and, one should get it checked so that they can be taken care of.

Once, these tests are done, it will be an eye opener, yes, we will be able to plan up the body transformation in an individualized and, professional manner. Also these results explain about the present position and, later on with time, we can get the parameters tested which are not in optimal range. This will be a guide for us to progress efficiently and, also monitor the progress.

All the above problems and, their remedies are discussed in detail in chapter 7.

CHAPTER 3

PHYSICAL SCREENING

Assessing the physical characteristics – Endurance, strength and, flexibility is really important. What we are as of now and, what the science says

Three aspects are really important for all the three above mentioned parameters –

a. Frequency – How many days in a week, the activity will be performed?

b. Intensity – What will be the intensity of the activity?

c. Time – What will be the duration of the activity?

Cardio-respiratory endurance

When it comes to endurance, or the cardiorespiratory endurance, it is really important to do it properly as it's the basics. The most effective way to burn fat.

Here lets discuss how fat is burned and, where does it melt away?

It's interesting!

Whenever we perform an activity, body needs fuel, this fuel is received from the burning of macros - Carbohydrates, fats and, proteins.

When we perform an activity in a prolonged manner or non stop manner at the desired heart rate, for the first 20 minute, the energy is provided by 80% of carbohydrates being processed,

Between 20 to 40 minutes, 50% fats and, 50% carbohydrates are being metabolized

Actually after 40 minutes 80% of fats are being burned

Now to increase the efficiency of the process, we need to understand, How and, where this fat melts away?

Fat molecules are made up of carbon, hydrogen and, oxygen. Just imagine they are attached with strings to each other, the more complex or entangled are the strings, the more difficult is to break them. In this manner only we define then as saturated, unsaturated and, poly unsaturated. Poly unsaturated are the weakest to break.

When these fat molecules break they form compounds carbon di oxide(CO_2) and, water (H_2O)

Water is discharged from the body in many forms, sweat is one of them (only the sweat, which comes when u performing an activity at target heart rate and, for a particular time period, dehydration is never fat loss) and, the carbon di oxide is emitted out during the breathing process while we work out. Here I would mention the more of fat is emitted out through the CO_2, we call it VO2 max – the amount of fat emitted out and, it can be calculated.

Now this 40 min to 1 hour cardio session is termed as low-intensity steady state cardio program. It definitely works, I have personally experienced it, also it doesn't need any particular skill and, a beginner also can manage it easily.

We may include fast walking, jogging, running, cycling, swimming and, many such activities.

(Other exercises will be discussed in Exercise Programming)

Pathways of energy metabolism

This is an important topic to understand, what is the source of energy for our activities

Cellular respiration is the process in which organisms break down glucose from food to create a usable form of energy that is called (ATP) Adenosine Tri Phosphate. When one of the phosphate groups break off, energy is released for all the cells to use. Different pathways of energy metabolism are as follows:

a) Aerobic Pathway – can only occur in the presence of oxygen, here the reactants glucose and, oxygen are turned into the products carbon dioxide, water and, ATP. Glycogen for aerobic metabolism is stored in muscle, liver and, blood. It is a slow process of recycling ATP, Fats and, proteins are also involved in aerobic pathway

b) Anaerobic Pathway – occurs when oxygen is not present in adequate amount. Glycogen fairly rapidly recycles ATP. It produces lactic acid and, It is the main energy system for exercise bouts ranging from 30sec to 3 minutes, high-intensity exercises with short intervals. It is active in long term, low intensity work outs

c) Creatine Phosphate Pathway – It is the process of recycling ATP from creatine phosphate, which is stored in muscle cells. It very rapidly recycles ATP. Usually 2-3 seconds of high-intensity work, Free ATP stores in muscle cells are depleted Then Creatine phosphate is involved to recycle ATP.

Let's take an example of swimming to understand the above energy pathways:

Creatine phosphate metabolism – diving and, turns – short distance with maximum intensity, swimming sets with short distances and, long intervals (a 10 second maximum intensity lap)

Anaerobic metabolism – high-intensity swimming sets with short rest intervals (4 sets of 30sec to 5 min high-intensity laps with short rest intervals

Aerobic Metabolism – low intensity, long distance, continuous laps (10min to 40 minutes continuous swimming)

Why the learning of these pathways important –

Now our target is fat loss, in that case, aerobic metabolism works the most for us, as it takes fat out of the fat cells and, burns it to produce energy for the muscles. It also burns up the available and, stored sugars (carbohydrates), so any excess won't be processed into fat. All the pathways will be used in the entire exercise program depending on our conditions and, goals.

Now, we understood that as far as endurance is concerned, what is the plan of action, Now what is important is to assess where we are?

Calculating the resting heart rate

As name suggest it's your pulse when we are not doing anything

I prefer checking it early morning just after bed

A Normal resting heart for adults ranges from 60 to 100 beats per minutes. Your resting heart rate is the heart pumping the lowest amount of blood you need because you are not exercising

Generally, a lower heart rate at rest implies more efficient heart function and, better cardio vascular fitness. For example a well trained athlete might have a normal resting heart rate closer to 40 beats per minute

The best places to find your pulse are the wrists, inside of the elbow or side of the neck.

Active people often have a lower resting heart rate because their heart muscle is in better condition and, doesn't need to work hard to maintain a steady beat. Your resting heart rate, when considered in the context of other markers such as blood pressure and, cholesterol, can help identify potential health problems as well as gauge your current health. Also a lower resting heart rate means a higher degree of fitness.

Now to start with, we will make a chart of our resting heart rate and, monitor it regularly and, make a weekly chart of the resting heart rate, its important. Regularly it will decrease with time when we will perform different activities in a continuous manner. Decreasing of the heart rate will be your first achievement as it is the basic sign of getting fit with time and, effort.

Calculating the target heart rate

In simple words its calculated as under

Maximum heart rate = 220 – age

Target heart rate = 60% to 80% of your maximum heart rate

(220-age) x 60% to 80%

I have seen people doing cardio activities in order to lose fat, in maximum cases, there are some common mistakes like:

1. People do their activity for just 10 – 20 minutes, but as mentioned above, if we are serious about body transformation and, want to lose fat, you have to do an activity or activities at a stretch from 40min to 60 min. Trust me the 10 – 20 min thing doesn't work as in this period 80% of carbohydrates are being burned.

2. People never take care of the heart rate, if you want to lose fat, then you have to reach your target heart rate and, then maintain it throughout the work out. I have seen people casually walking in parks, on treadmills, or having fun while cycling etc, trust me these will never work.

3. Nowadays group sessions are really in practice, but I have seen there are breaks, in this case no what is the intensity of the class is, the rhythm or the elevation drops, that is also a disturbing factor. I always remember doing jumping jacks or high speed on spot run while I used to attend group activities at the time of break in classes.

4. One thing I have seen is short term high-intensity work outs

In this case, just imagine someone doing a sprint for 2 min or 5 min on treadmill, here the metabolism in action during exercise to provide the fuel is basically anaerobic (as discussed in the energy pathways) and, in this case the fat loss will not be to that extent.

Most effective way to do cardiovascular training

Let's assume a person of age 30

Let's calculate his maximum heart rate first – 220 minus 30 = 190

Now if he is a beginner then he should start his work out at 60% of his maximum heart rate.

That means – 190 x 60% (60% of his efficiency) = 114

His target heart rate is 114 and, it should be maintained through out the activity.

You can start maintaining heart rate at 50% - 60% initially and, then gradually with time and, as your endurance will increase you will be able to increase the intensity to 80%.

I must mention here, it's a continued effort and, it will take time, also not one or two work outs will give results, As per the designed schedule whether its twice a week or five days a week depending on your fat percentage you have to do it your endurance work outs. Initially it will be a tough job but with time u will be able to do it. You can choose the activity as per your comfort and, start doing it as long as you can do it.

Let's assume walking, if I say the final target is doing 5km in 40 min, then initially you can do it for just 20 minutes and, see your endurance, then with time make it 40 minutes irrespective of the distance, then third stage try increase your speed and, cover as much distance as possible and, record it. With time you will achieve your target and, when you are comfortable you can increase your time upto 60 minutes.

Gradually you will start losing fat and, also your endurance will help you in your daily activities, sleep patterns, blood circulation, also it will increase your strength and, endurance in your other work outs which will help you achieve your goals.

Now considering the above two aspects Energy Pathways and, the target heart rate:

We conclude that the best form of endurance work outs to lose maximum fat is

Doing a continuous activity for more than 40 minutes at the target heart rate and, the no of times you have to do it in a week will depend on your fat percentage.

It is really important to understand your present position

I called it Self Assesment

Many a times I have seen people following the practice of Too Soon Too Fast.

Trust me it never works, What happens is one fine day you realized you have gained weight, then next morning you go for a rigorous walk of 60 minutes, without thinking about your present condition.

The second day, your full body is paining, the third day somehow you went for walking in pain, you again did it for 50 minutes and, come back, the fourth day pain become severe, and, fifth day are not able to do your daily activities and, the sixth day you give up and, for next seven days you were having pain killers and, applying ointments.

In this case, the approach should be

Day 1 – Day 3 -20 minutes brisk walk and, stretching

Day 4 – Day 7 – 40 minutes walking and, stretching

Then gradually the speed and, time can be increased with proper stretching and, cool down

When we talk in terms of theory

Your present endurance can be checked by checking that how fast your heart rate increases while progressing in an activity and, how fast it comes down when you have finished an activity.

It's really important to understand this pattern or we wont be able to reach our goals and, will be either injured or disheartened.

Cardio respiratory fitness assessment or monitoring exercise intensity

Of the numerous methods of monitoring exercise intensity, some have been standardized and, recommended.

The method you choose will depend on your exercise program and, level of fitness.

The following are the methods of monitoring exercise intensity:

1. ***Percentage of maximal heart rate*** – This method of monitoring intensity of exercise calculates the exercise heart rate as a percentage of maximal heart rate.

   Training heart rate = maximal measured or predicted heart rate x 60% to 90% (desired percent of maximal HR)

   For example

   A 40 year old man for whom an intensity of 70% of maximal heart rate is desired

   220 – Age = 220-40 = 180 (predicted maximum heart rate)

   180 x 70% (70 % exercise intensity)

   126 = Exercise heart rate

   In this way you can definitely check your intensity with time and, progress gradually for maximum results.

2. ***Rating of Perceived exertion*** – Exercise intensity also can be measured by assigning a numerical value (0 to 10) to subjective feelings of exercise exertion. Rating of perceived exertion takes into account all that the exercising person is perceiving in terms of exercise fatigue, including psychological, muscoskeletal and, environmental factors. The RPE response also correlates well with cardiorespiratory and, metabolic factors such as heart rate, breathing rate, oxygen consumption and, overall fatigue. This level of perceived physical effort is assigning a rating in the following scale

Scale is like

0 – Feeling nothing at all

1 – very weak

2 – weak

3 – moderate

4 – somewhat strong

5 – strong

6

7 very strong

8

9

10 – very very strong, maximal

An RPE of 8 would correspond to about 80% of maximal heart rate. Accordingly you can calculate the intensity and, progress each time you work out.

The Talk Test Method – Another means of evaluating the intensity of exercise is the talk test. Like the RPE method, the talk test is subjective, but it is quite useful in determining the comfort zone of aerobic intensity. You should be able to breathe comfortably and, rhythmically throughout all phases of a work out to ensure a safe and, comfortable level of exercise, especially for those just beginning an exercise program. Those who progress to higher functional capacities and, higher level work outs may find this technique somewhat conservative, especially at intensities greater 80% of functional capacity.

Strength assesment

Importance of muscle mass in body transformation

When we are looking forward to body Transformation, In initial stages your fat percentage is really high.

Here I will take an example

Let's assume two people A and, B with same weight, 80 kg

A has 70 kg muscle weight and, 10 kg fat weight

B has 60 kg muscle weight and, 20 kg fat weight

1. The first thing which comes into picture is the look. Just imagine 1kg of iron and, 1 kg of cotton. Which one will look thin or which one will take less space, obviously 1 kg of iron.

    In this case also A will look much tighter, toned and, lean, though they have equal bodyweight.

2. M FOR MUSCLE, M FOR METABOLISM – A has better metabolism than B and, will be less prone to diabetes, obesity and, other related issues.

    One of the most important functions of muscle in metabolic health is their ability to store glucose (carbohydrates) as glycogen. They then use this stored glycogen as fuel every time you need to move. This makes muscle a critical player in an overall healthy metabolism, and, also increases insulin sensitivity and, protects against insulin resistance. Also in helping your body using carbohydrates this way, muscle mass is ultimately protective and, metabolic syndrome and, diabetes, which are really just diseases of inadequate carbohydrate metabolism as the unused glycogen is stored in the form of triglycerides and, then as stored fat.

3. A with healthy muscles will move freely with a stronger body, also he will be able to perform his daily activities in a better manner. Strong muscles also help to keep joints in good shape. If the muscles around the knee joint, for example, get weak, possibility of injury increases.

Apart from the basic functions, Muscle count is the most important aspect in Body Transformation. We can achieve our goals faster and, in a smooth injury free manner, if we take care of our muscle count from the very beginning. I always say an athlete's life is the most difficult, he has to eat less to cut down fat and, at the same time he has to eat more to maintain or increase the muscle weight. It's not the calories, it's the difference between the good and, the bad calories that we need to understand and, at the same time the amount of strength based activities that need to be performed.

Trust me when you lose fat and, build muscles at the same time you actually get fit and, you look fitter. That's what actually is Body Transformation.

Difference between fat loss and, muscle loss

If I ask any one what is your goal, the person answers I want to lose fat, but when I start an exercise program I say I want to gain muscle strength.

I will give an example. Let's assume a boy whose weight is 70 kgs and, fat percentage is 30%

In this case the muscle weight is 49kgs and, fat weight is 21 kgs

Now I give three examples –

Case 1 - One is to reduce the fat weight, lets assume it came down to 15kgs and, total weight is now 64 kgs then the fat percentage will be approx 23%.

Case 2 - Second is we increase the muscle weight by 3 kgs and, decrease the fat by 3 kgs, in that case the overall weight remains the same and, now the muscle weight is 52kgs and, the fat weight is 18kgs and, the fat percentage is approximately 25.7 %

Case 3 - Third is, the fat weight is reduced by 2 kgs and, the muscle weight is also reduced by 4kgs. Now the muscle weight is 45kgs, fat weight is 19 kgs and, now the fat percentage is 29.7%

Now, as we have discussed earlier, total weight is the sum of muscle weight and, fat weight.

Muscle weight is the good weight we have, and, its never preferred to lose muscle weight.

In all three cases the person has lost 6kgs of overall weight but

In case 1 the muscle weight is constant, that means muscle weight has been maintained by strength training and, proper nutrition

In case 2 the muscle weight is reduced with the fat weight, which is not good, I may say strength training is there but nutrition is lacking

In case 3, as you can see after losing 6kgs the fat percentage is still the same, because the person has reduced more of muscle mass. In this case, probably the nutrition and, strength training both are lacking.

Frankly speaking, Case 3 is mostly seen around. The day we think about Body Transformation, our first criteria and, concern is losing weight anyhow, just to satisfy the weighing scale and, nothing else.

We do not do strength-based activities and, also do not take care of our nutrition, that's why what we lose is only muscles and, water. Here I ll mention that what a person does, they start rigorous work outs and, stop having balanced diet. What happens, in this case, the body is not able to maintain the muscle mass and, it drops drastically. Let me tell you that fat is the body's reserve for energy. It is not released easily.

Let me give an example:

You have a current account and, fixed deposits, in your daily life you always rely on your current accounts and, in case of emergency only you will use your fixed deposits.

It's the same with the body, fats are body's fixed deposits, they are never used easily, u need to have patience, if you apply the strategy Too Fast Too Soon, you will end up losing muscles and, nothing else. Also the case 3 state is known as the catabolic or the negative state for the body and, gradually it weakens us from inside, which is not good.

Also this is the reason why people losing weight are not able to maintain the lost weight, because infact they have lost muscle weight and, some water, the fat is still there, the moment they get back to their original daily routine the weight bounces back. Here I will definitely say, mostly the practice is to reduce taking carbohydrates and, salt in diet, these two hold the water inside the body, the moment we stop these two as per certain popular diets, we suddenly lose weight, but let me re insist it's not fat that you have lost, its just water and, muscles, that's all, the moment you will go back to your normal diet the weight will bounce back. Also in this case, the muscle weakens and, the people get body pains and, they are not able to carry on with their work outs and, hence they give up.

We need to get stronger when we are doing body transformation, remember our goal is to lose the fat weight the bad weight, not the good weight the muscle weight.

This shows that taking care of the muscle weight is very important.

Strength testing procedures without any equipment

In this case also personal assessment is important, what is your present position

Strength is the ability to carry out work against a resistance, the maximum force that can be generated depends on the size and, the number of muscles involved or I should say muscle fibres called into action

In this case, there is no single test for strength, each strength test is specific to the action and, muscle group being tested.

Here is a list of strength and, strength endurance tests

Strength Fitnes Tests without any equipment

1. Strength test for Upper Body

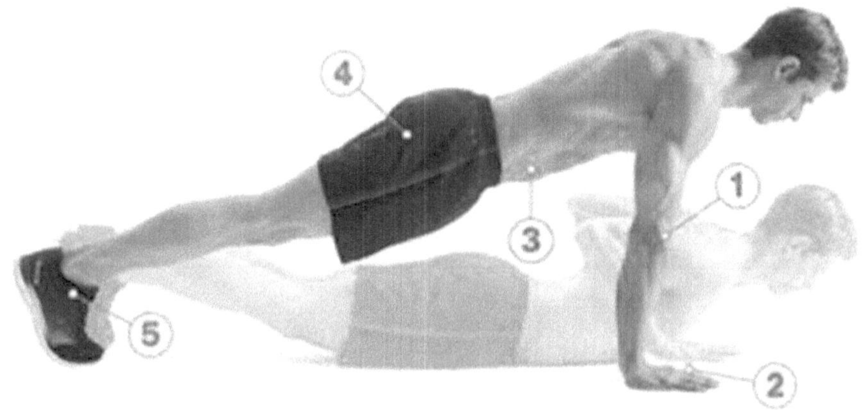

Pushups

a) Push UP Test – How many push-ups you can do?

Men should use the standard pushup position with only the hands and, the toes touching the floor in the starting position. Women has the additional option of using the bent knee position.

Lower the chest down towards the floor, always do the same level each time, either till our elbows are at the right angles or your chest touches the ground.

Do as many pushups as possible until exhaustion, count them and, use the chart to find how you rate

Men						
Age	17-19	20-29	30-39	40-49	50-59	60-65
Excellent	>56	>47	>41	>34	>31	>30
Good	47-56	39-47	34-41	28-34	25-31	24-30
Above Average	35-46	30-39	25-33	21-28	18-24	17-23
Average	19-34	17-29	13-24	11-20	9-17	6-16
Below Average	11-18	10-16	8-12	6-10	5-8	3-5
Poor	4-10	4-9	2-7	1-5	1-4	1-2
Very Poor	<4	<4	<2	0	0	0
Women						
Age	17-19	20-29	30-39	40-49	50-59	60-65
Excellent	>35	>36	>37	>31	>25	>23
Good	27-35	30-36	30-37	25-31	21-25	19-23
Above Average	21-27	23-29	22-30	18-24	15-20	13-18
Average	11-20	12-22	10-21	8-17	7-14	5-12
Below Average	6-10	7-11	5-9	4-7	3-6	2-4
Poor	2-5	2-6	1-4	1-3	1-2	1
Very Poor	<2	<1	0	0	0	0

Remember, these tests scores are based on doing the tests as described, and, may not be accurate if the test is modified. Don't worry too much how much you rate, just try and, improve your own score, and, keep them the same way each time.

b) Pull Up Test –

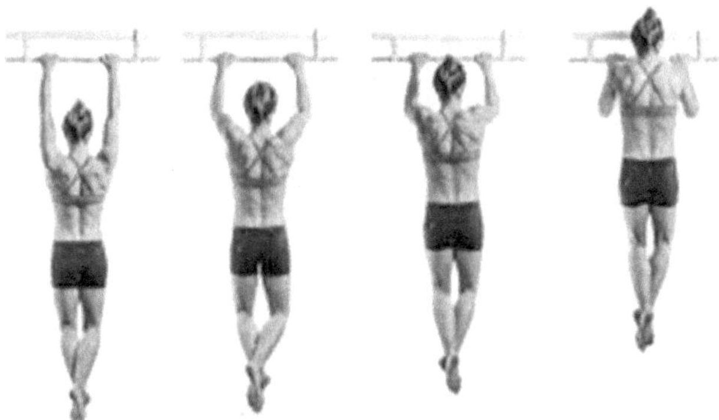

Pullups

The Pull up test also called the chin-up test is widely used as a measure of upper body strength. You should grasp an overhead bar and, pull up the body so the chin raises above the bar, then returns to arms fully extended position.

In this case you can use the over hand grip or the under hand grip. The totalnumber of correctly completed pull ups is recorder. The type of grip should also be recorded with the results.

Initially you may find it difficult, but gradually with time you will be able to do it when the muscle strength increases with proper training and, nutrition.

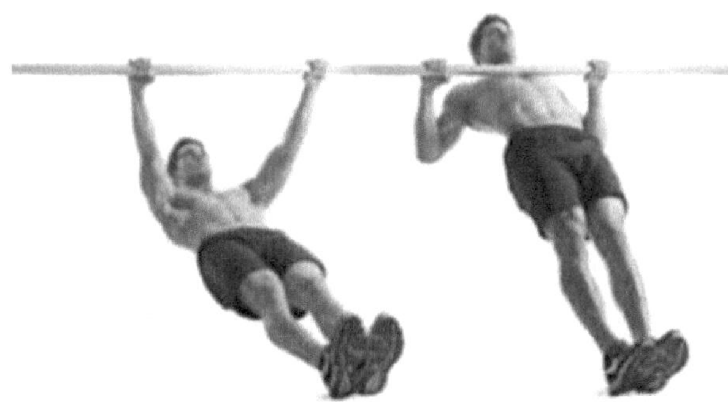

Horizontal pullup

One variation to this pull up test is Horizontal Pull up Test: It is easier than the Pull up Test, as the whole bodyweight does not need to be pulled up. You need to set the horizontal bar so that when the arms are fully extended, the upper body is off the ground. You have to grip slightly wider than shoulder using an overhand or underhand grip. The feet are placed flat on the ground so that knees are bent at 90 degrees angle, to increase the intensity you can keep the feet on a chair also. Now pull your body upwards until the chest touches the bar and, then lower yourself till the arsm are fully extended. Repeat as many times as u can and, record the transactions.

c)   Dips to the front and, Dips behind the back – This test measures upper body strength.

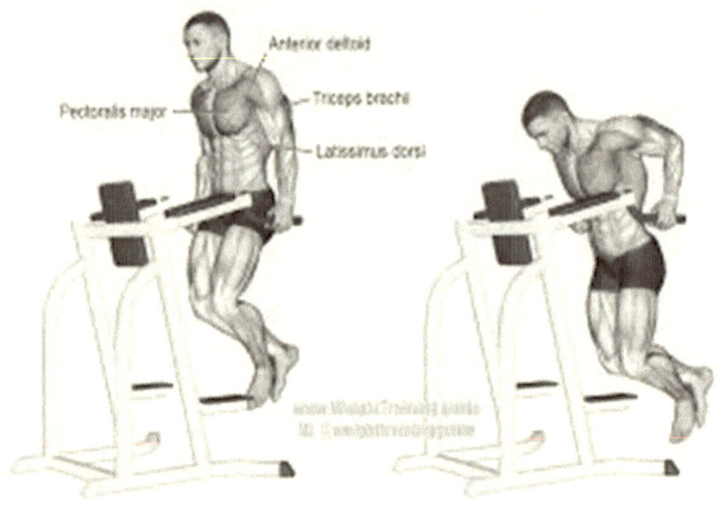

Dips

For Dips to the front you need parallel bars or two parallel hard surfaces having gap in between of appropriate height. You start in the up position, with the arms and, elbows fully locked. One complete dip is performed by bending the arms and, lowering the body until the elbows are bent to atleast a right angle and, then pushing to the starting position.

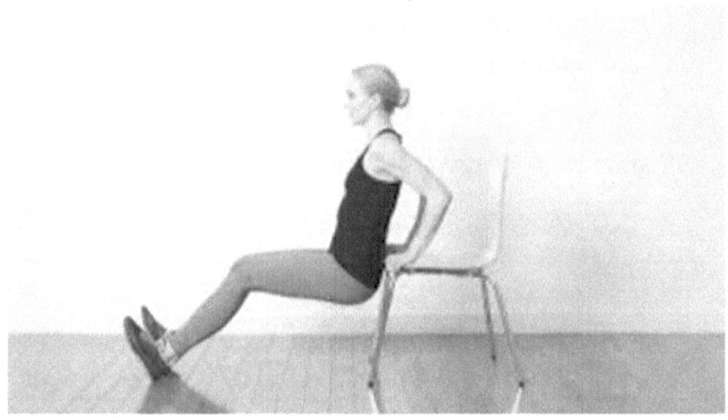

Dips behind the back

For Dips behind the back, you need a hard surface like a chair or a sofa, just sit on the surface, place your hands on the chair towards the side and, lift your body up and, then go down so as to your seat muscle approaching the floor till your elbows are at right angle

You may record the transactions

2. Strength Fitness Test For Lower Body –

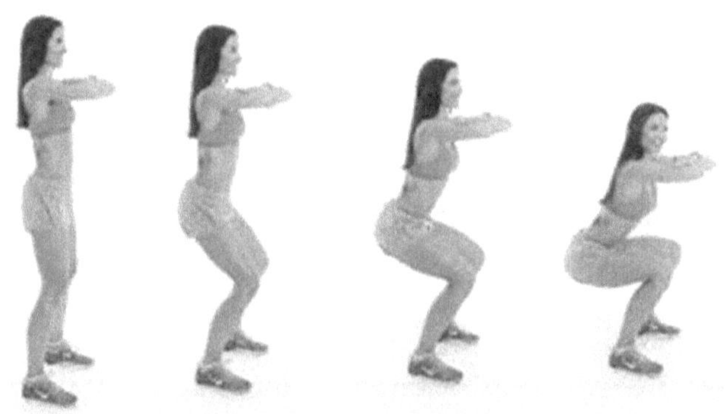

Squats

a)   Squats - How many squats you can do?

Stand in front of a chair or bench with your feet shoulder apart, facing away from it. Your hands can be sideways, crossed on chest or behind the neck. Squat down and, lightly touch the chair before standing back up. A good sized chair is one that makes your knees at right angle when you are sitting.

Compare your results to the tables below

Men					
Age	20-29	30-39	40-49	50-59	60-65
Excellent	>34	>32	>29	>26	>23
Good	33	30	27	24	22
Above Average	30	27	24	22	18
Average	27	24	21	18	15
Below Average	24	21	18	15	12
Poor	21	18	15	12	9
Very Poor	<15	<12	<10	<7	<5
Women					
Age	20-29	30-39	40-49	50-59	60-65
Excellent	>29	>26	>23	>20	>17
Good	28	25	22	19	16
Above Average	25	22	19	16	13
Average	21	18	15	12	9
Below Average	17	14	11	8	5
Poor	15	12	9	6	3
Very Poor	<14	<11	<8	<5	<3

Initially you shouldn't worry too much about how you rate, just try to improve your own score with time, diet and, training. These figures can just be guide.

3) Core strength Tests without Equipment – Abdominal muscle strength and, endurance is important for core stability and, back support.

a)   Sit Up Test –

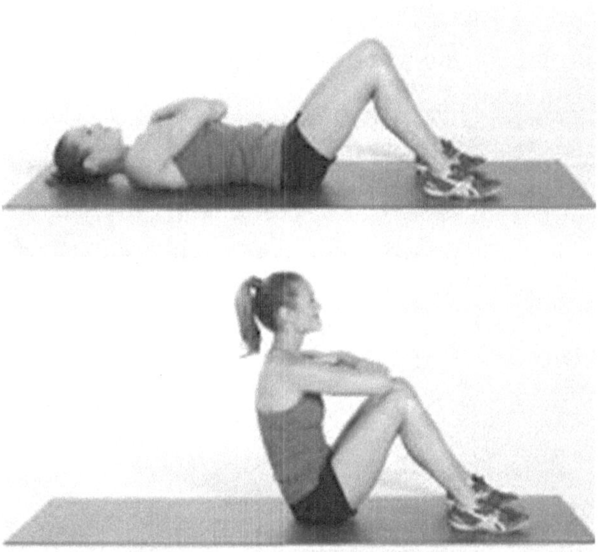

Sit up test

This Sit Up Test measures the strength and, endurance of the muscles. How many sit ups you can do at different levels

You lie on your back, with the knees at right angle and, feet flat on the floor. Now you perform one complete sit up for each level in the prescribed manner as below, starting from level 1

Level 1 – Poor - Arms extended, you curl up so that the wrist reach the knees

Level 2 – Fair - Arms extended, you curl up so that elbows reach the knees

Level 3 – Average - Arms held together across abdominals, curl up so that chest touches the thighs

Level 4 – Good - Arms held across the chest, holding shoulders, curl up so that forearm touches the thighs

Level 5 – Very Good - Hands held behind the head, curl up so that chest touches thighs

Level 6 – Excellent - As per level 5, with a 2 kg water bottle or dumbbell held behind head, chest touching thighs

Level 7 – Elite - As per level 5, with a 5 kg dumbbell held behind head, chest touching thighs

Start from level 1 and, check your strength, Gradually with practice and, consistency you will be able to reach higher levels.

b)   Plank Test –

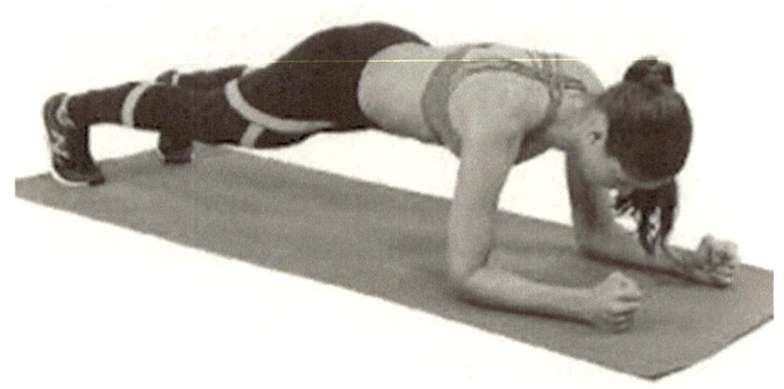

Plank

The plank test measures the control the control and, endurance of the core stabilizing muscles.

The aim of this test is to hold an elevated position as long as possible. Start with the upper body supports off the ground by the elbows and, forearms, and, the legs straight with the weight taken by the toes. The hip is lifted off the floor creating a straight line from head to toe. Then start the stopwatch.

The scoring is the total time completed

Rating	Time
Excellent	>6minutes
Very Good	4-6 minutes
Above Average	2-4 minutes
Average	1-2 minutes
Below Average	30-60 seconds
Poor	15-30 seconds
Very poor	<15 seconds

One variation for this test is the Side Plank Test

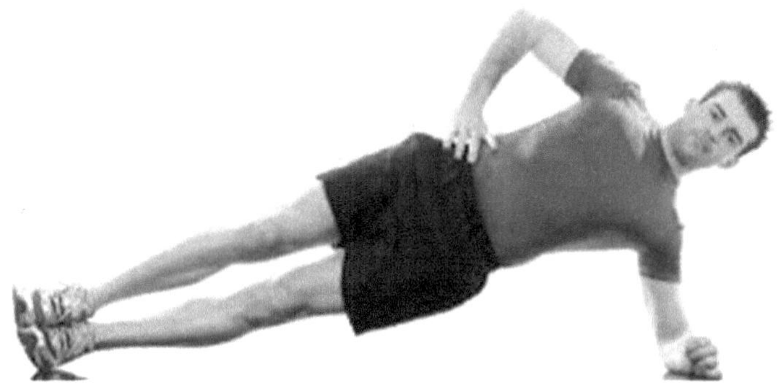

Side Plank

This test measures the control of the control and, endurance of the lateral core stabilizing muscles

The aim is to hold an elevated position as long as possible

Lie on the right side or left side, whichever comfortable, the upper body supported off the ground by the elbow and, forearm, the legs are straight, one over the other. The hip is lifted off the floor so that the elbow and, feet support the body, creating a staright line from head to toe.

Then the stopwatch is started.

The scoring is the total time completed

Rating	Time(seconds)
Excellent	>90
Good	75 to 90
Average	60 to 75
Poor	<60

c) Straight Leg lift Abdominal Strength Test –

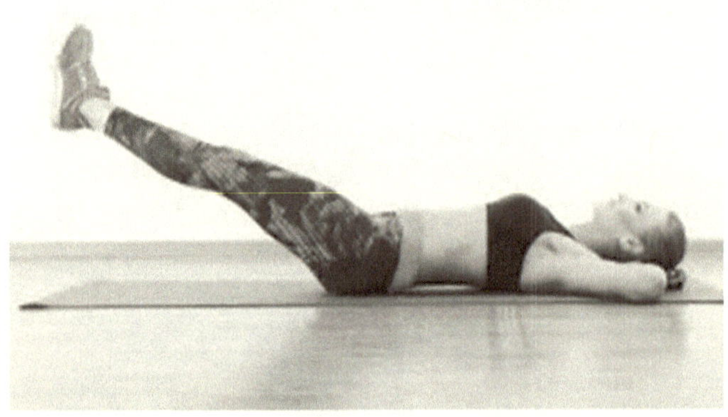

The purpose of this test is to estimate the degree of abdominal strength. This test is important to conduct as poor abdominal muscle strength can cause poor posture leading ti lower back pain.

Lie on the floor on your back, bend your legs and, raise them to 90 degrees, now place one of your hand under your lower back. Now contract your abdominal muscle to press your arm and, gradually without bending the knees, slowly lower both legs until the pressure on the hand behind the back disappears. The lowest angle observed as the pressure is taken off is the measurement of your abdominal strength.

The score is the angle of the legs in degrees from the floor.

Please compare the score with the below chart –

Angle(Degrees)	Rating
90	very poor, starting position
75	poor
60	below average
45	average
30	above average
15	good
5	excellent

The muscles play a major role in the effort to maintain the position of the lower back and, pelvis during the leg lowering movement are the rectus abdominis and, external oblique muscles.

d) Back Strength Test

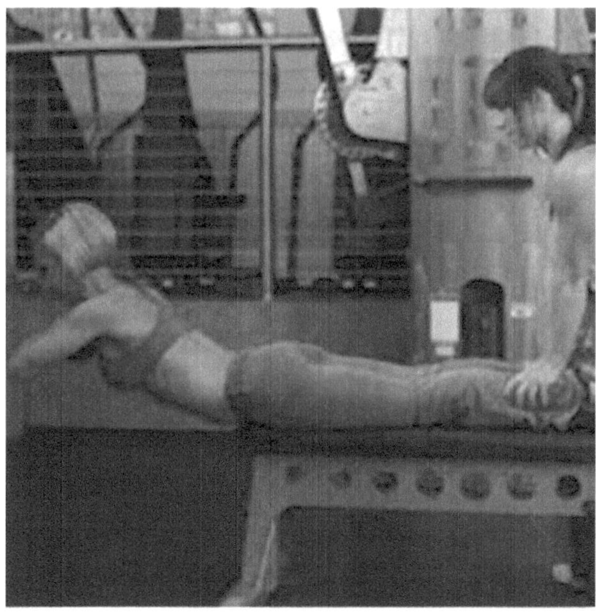

Hyper extension test

The isometric back strength test is a measure of the strength of the muscles of the lower back, which is important in core stability and, for preventing lower back pain.

Lie face down on a bench, with your upper body from the waist hanging over the end of the bench, ask someone to hold your ankles and, your arms are behind your neck. When ready, bring your body up to the horizontal position and, hold this for a set period (eg. – 30 to 45 seconds.

This test will assess your back strength.

Here it is important to mention, for the people who are already in the fitness industry and, have been doing work out from some time, and, also are going to fitness club should also assess their strength by the following strength tests

Strength testing procedures with equipments

These tests are known as 1-RM, one repetition maximum tests.

The one repetition maximum tests is a measure of the maximal weight a person can lift with one repetition. It iss a popular method of measuring isotonic muscle strength. Below is a description of the procedure of the repetition max test

It is important to reach the maximum weight carrying capacity without prior fatiguing the muscles. After a warm up, choose a weight that is achievable. Then after rest, increase the weight and, do again. Keep gradually increasing the weight till you can do only one repetition with the weight.

The maximum weight lifted is recorded, the sequence of the lifts should also be recorded as these can be used in future when we are again conducting the test for determining the lift to attempt.

Primarily 1 RM Test is conducted in the following exercises

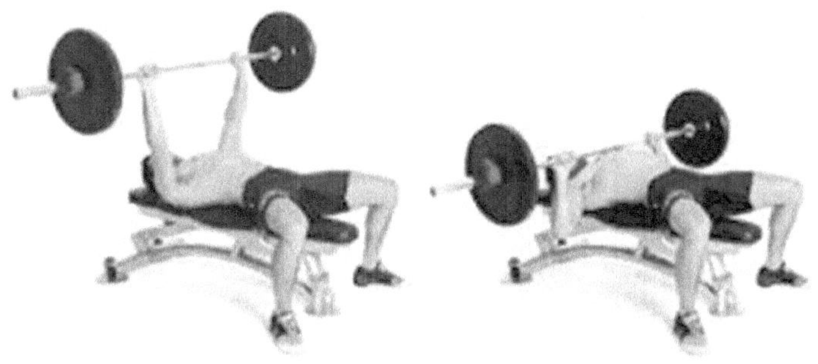

Bench Press

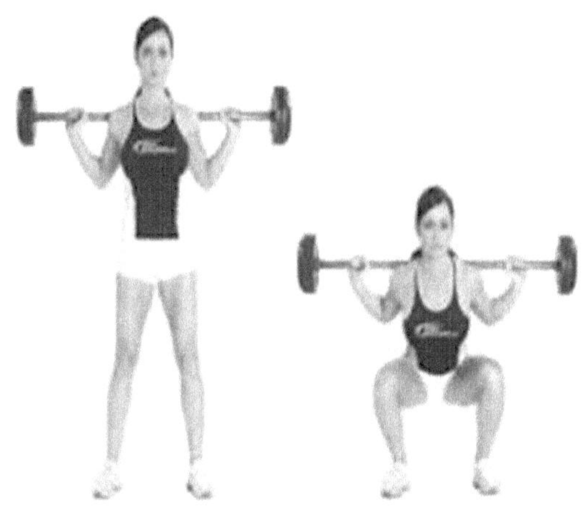

Weighted Squats

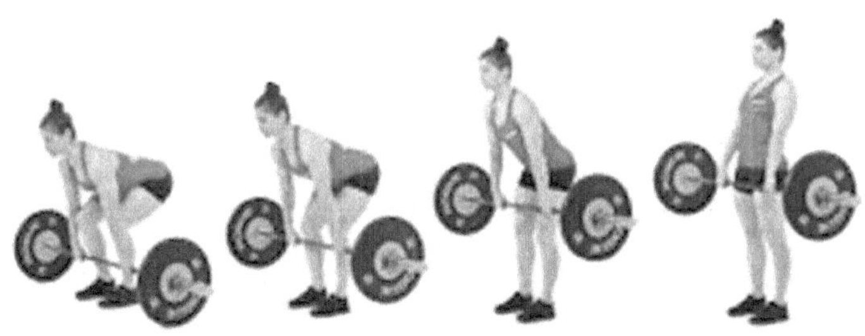

Deadlift

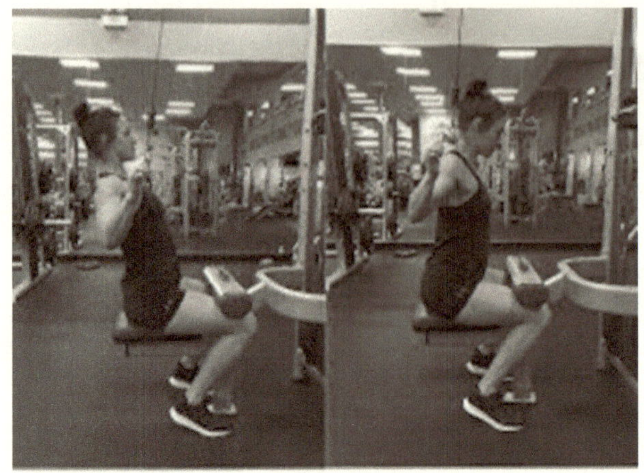

Lat pull down

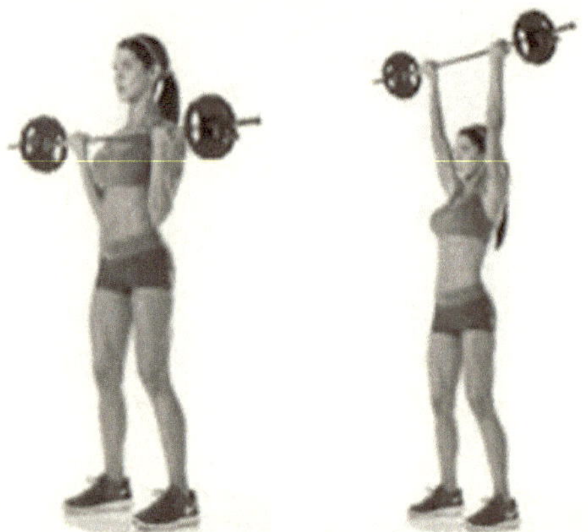

Shoulder press

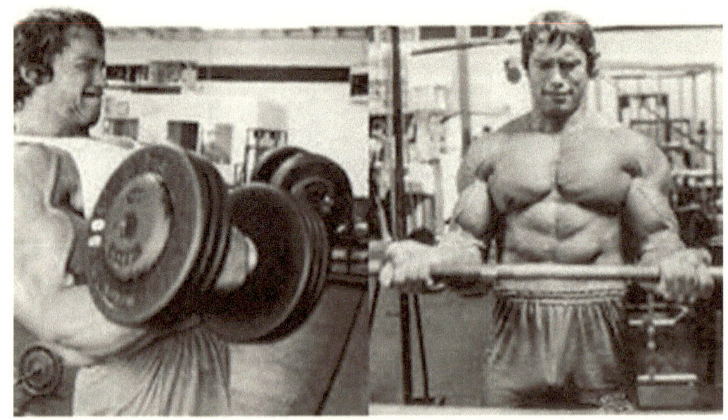

Bicep Curls

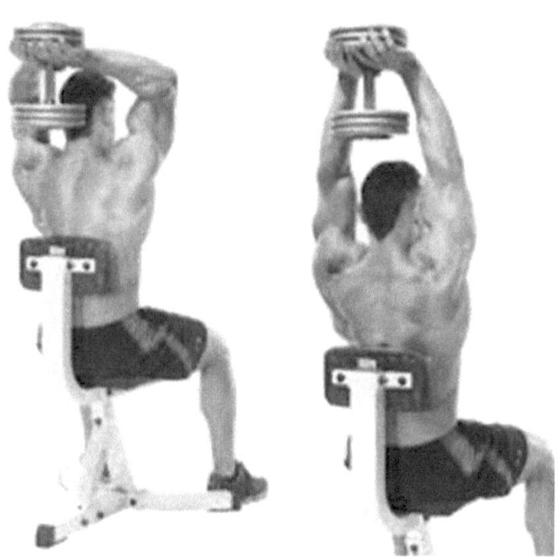

Tricep Extensions

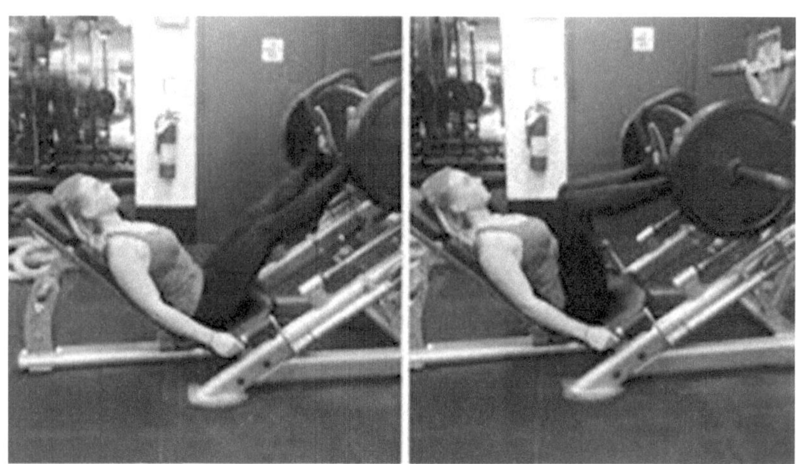

Leg Press

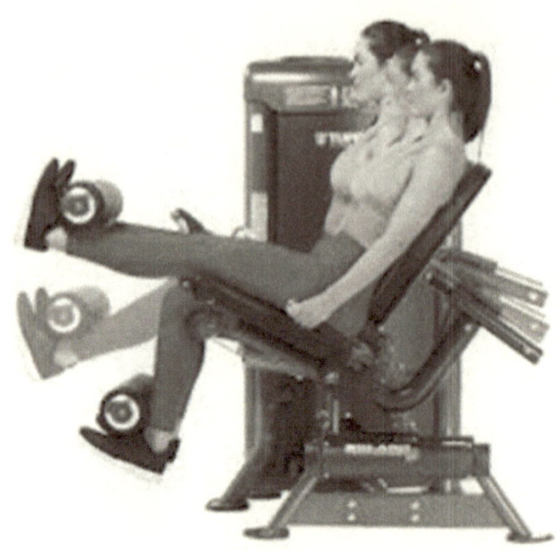

Leg Extensions

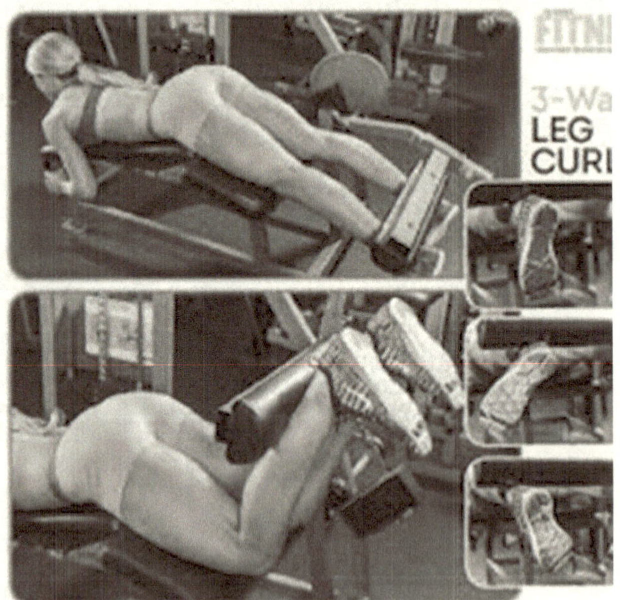

Leg curls

Bench press, Squats, Deadlift, Lat Pull Downs, Shoulder presses, bicep curl, tricep extensions, leg presses, leg curls and, extensions

You should take this test every fortnight or once in a month for all the exercises mentioned above to test your muscle strength and, power. This ensures that with due course of time our muscle weight is increasing or is maintained throughout the body transformation.

In fact all the above mentioned tests, without equipment and, with equipment should be taken regularly.

Flexibility assessment

Importance and, benefits of flexibility in body transformation

Now we have understood the importance of strength and, endurance in Body Transformation, let's discuss about Flexibility.

Most people take part in aerobic activities to improve their cardiovascular endurance and, burn fat. People weight train to maintain lean muscle tissue and, build strength.

These two elements are considered to be the most important? Right?

Whenever we talk about Body Transformation, Flexibility is a topic which is always under estimated and, ignored. In fact flexibility is a term which plays the most essential role. In lay man terms flexibility is the range of motion in a joint or series of joints, and, length in muscles that cross the joints to induce a bending movement or motion. It varies from person to person but it can be increased by exercise.

Some people are naturally more flexible. Flexibility is primarily due to one's genetics, gender, age, body shape, but I insist It depends on the level of physical activity, also as people grow older, they tend to lose flexibility. The less active you are, the less flexible you are likely to be.

In our daily life, we never emphasize on flexibility or stretching, In case when we are concerned with our health or fitness, the maximum we take care is about our diet or focus on work out routines.

Here I would mention, for someone who is not used to regular work outs, or is just starting with an exercise program the best way to start is to inform your body that you will be starting with something new.

Just understand, whenever we start a work out what are the few things that happen

1. The heart has to pump more blood in the particular area, like if we start with a walk, what happens, the leg muscles needs more blood or more oxygen, more nutrients to work for the time being you are walking. It's an unusual activity for your body, It has to get accustomed with the routine, which will take time. Let's give time to ourselves.

2. When you walk more than usual, the involved group of muscles, legs, have to work more, which the legs are not used to. In this case various muscle fibers and, joints come into play and, in starting they can be overworked or I can say over trained which may result in fatigue and, at times pain too.

In both the cases, it can disturb the course of action and, you may not be able to carry your Body Transformation for long.

The best way is to start gradually. Also I would mention, whether you are in any stage of your Body Transformation, flexibility routines should be a part of your program, it prepare your body for something rigorous and, unusual, and, also at the same time relaxes and, rejuvenates your body from the hard work out routines and, helps in removing the lactic acid also.

Here are certain benefits of practicing flexibility routines regularly –

1. Once you develop strength and, flexibility in your body you will be able to withstand more physical stress, also you will get rid of any muscle imbalances, which reduces the chance of getting injured during your work outs. In this case we strengthen the underactive muscles and, stretch the overactive or the stiff or tight ones.

2. Your body is likely to feel better overall once you work on lengthening and, opening your muscles. When your muscles are lose and, less tense, body pain will be much lesser.

3. As mentioned above with regular stretching routines, lactic acid formation will be much less, leading to relaxed muscles and, the pains will be reduced.

4. When you focus on increasing muscular flexibility your posture is likely to improve. Also with an increased range of motion it is easier to perform many activities.

5. When we practice stretching regularly, the lose or the flabby skin gets toned up.

6. A very important point I would like to mention, in certain cases, I have seen, if one or the other joint is injured or is not allowing intense work outs, in that case stretching exercises really helps to work out and, tone up the muscles around that joint.

Types of stretching

1. Static Stretching – It's the most common and, is executed by extending the targeted muscle group to its maximum point for 30 seconds or more. Her when you apply the added force its known as active static stretching and, when the force is added by a device or a partner its known as passive static stretching.

2. Dynamic Stretching – Its uses primarily for athletic drills and, utilizes repeated bouncing movement to stretch the target muscle group. It should be safely performed from low velocity to high velocity and, preceded by static stretching.

3. Active Isolated Stretching – It is performed for several sets with a specific number of repetitions. Much like a strength training regime. Here we stay at a point just for few seconds and, It is performed repeatedly for several repetitions, each time exceeding the previous point of resistance by a few degrees.

4. PNF – Proprioceptive Neuromuscular Facilitation - It usually employs the use of a partner to provide resistance against the isometric contraction and, then later to passively take the joint through its increased range of motion.

Now when we know the benefits and, types of stretching lets test ourselves before starting any kind of flexibility training or stretching program as without assessing our present position it can lead to short term and, long term injuries.

Flexibility testing procedures

1. Sit and, Reach Flexibility Test –

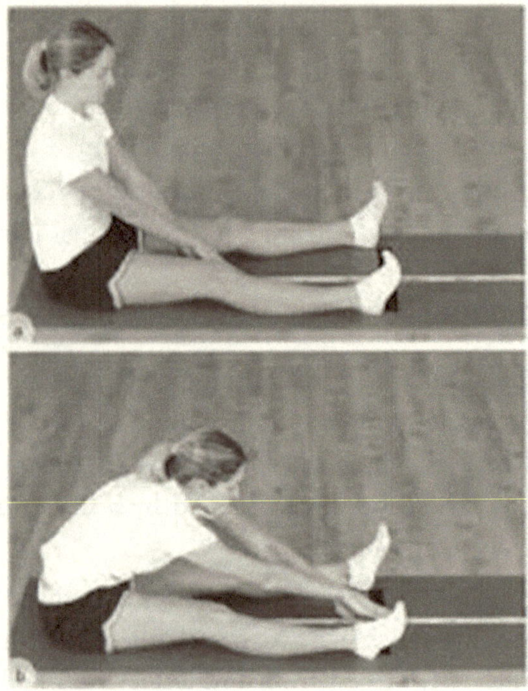

Sit and reach flexibility test

The sit and, reach test is a common measure of flexibility, and, specifically measures the flexibility of the lower back and, hamstring muscles.

This test involves sitting on the floor without shoes with legs stretched out straight ahead.

The most logical measure is to use the level of the feet as recording zero, now any measure that does not reach the toes is and, any reach past the toes is positive.

2. Toe Touch Test –

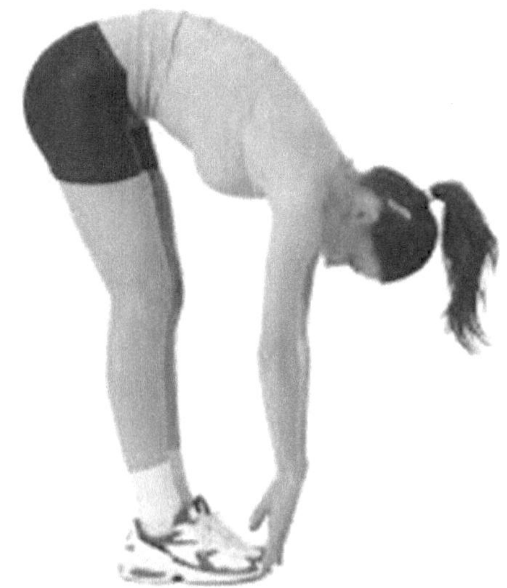

Toe touch test

This test also measures the flexibility of the lower back and, hamstring muscles. You stand erect, bare-footed, and, with feet slightly apart. Then bend at the waist to lean slowly forward to attempt to touch the ground with finger-tips, the handle flat with the finger outstretched without bouncing and, jerking. The knees must be kept straight.

3. Groin Flexibility –

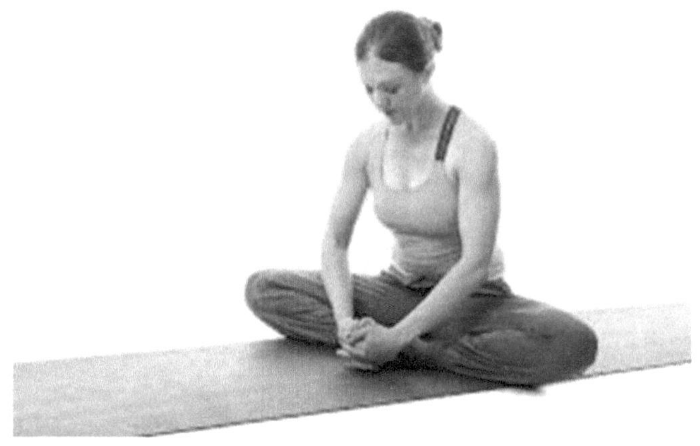

Groin Flexibility

Sit on the floor with your knees bent, and, your feet flat on the floor and, legs together. Let your knees drop sideways as far as possible keeping your feet together. The soles of the feet should be together and, facing each other. Grab hold on to your aankles with both hands and, pull them as close to your body as possible. Measure the distance from your heels to your groin. Use the table mentioned below –

Excellent   5cm

Very Good   10cm

Good   15cm

Fair   20cm

Poor   25cm

4. Lateral side Bending Flexibility Tests –

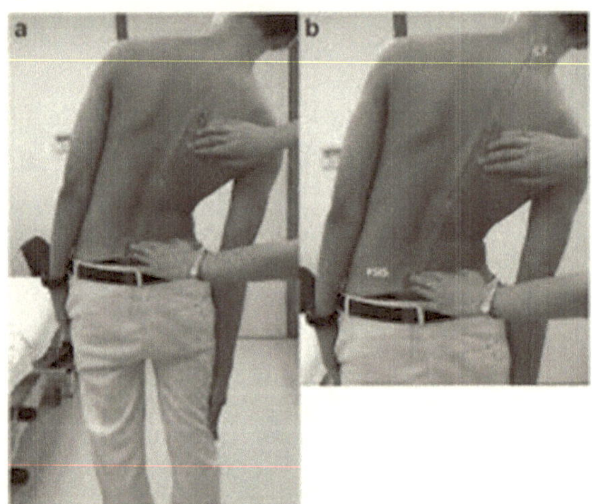

Lateral side bending flexibility test

It is a measure of trunk flexibility. It measures the average range of movement in lateral flexion of the thoracic, lumbar spine and, pelvis. Please stand upright against a wall on two parallel lines at right angles to the wall and, 15cm apart. The arms are held straight against the sides of the body. The level of the middle finger on each side is marked with a horizontal line on the side of the thigh. Then slowly bend sideways as far as possible while maintaining contact between the back and, the wall. The distance between the first and, last position of the middle finger is recorded.

5. Trunk Rotation Test –

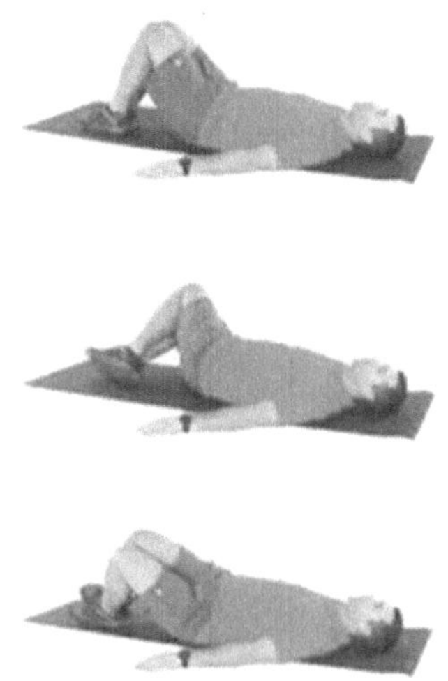

Trunk rotation flexibility test

It is to measure trunk and, shoulder flexibility which is important for injury prevention. Make a vertical line on the wall. Stand with your back to the wall directly in front of the line, with your shoulder width apart. Extend your arms directly in front of you, twist your trunk to your right and, touch the wall behind with the fingertips. You can move shoulder, hips and, knees as far as feet are stationary. Mark the position where your fingertips touch the wall and, measure the distance from the line. Repeat for the left side.

Use the table mentioned below –

Excellent	20cm
Very Good	15cm
Good	10cm
Fair	5cm
Poor	0cm

Shoulder Stretch Test –

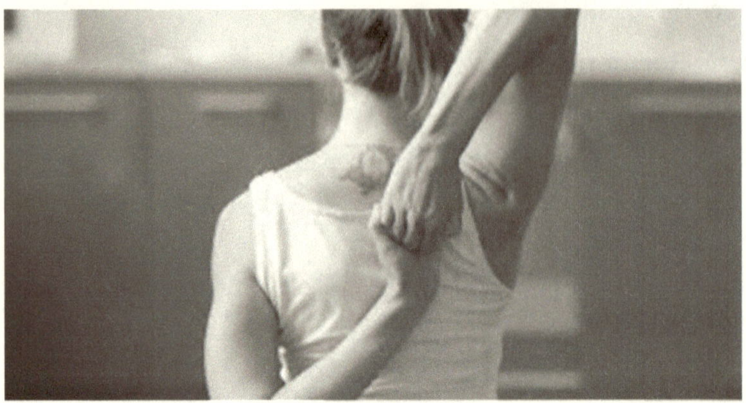

Shoulder stretch test

This test is a simple flexibility test to determine if the hands can be brought together behind the back. In standing position, place one hand behind the head and, back over the shoulder, and, reach as far as possible down the middle of your back, your palm touching your body and, the fingers directed downwards. Place the other arm behind your back, palm facing outward and, fingers upward and, reach up as far as possible attempting to touch the fingers of each hand.

6. Flexibility test for Hip Rotators –

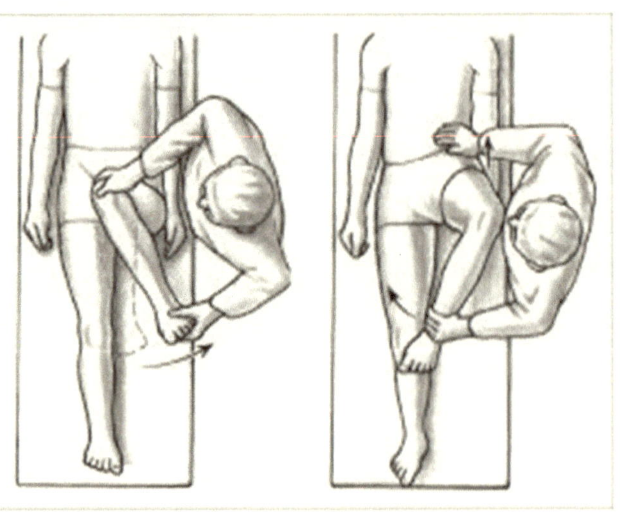

Hip Rotation test

Lie on your back, with the left foot on the ground and, right ankle resting gently on top of the left knee. Lift the left leg up off the ground and, try to reach for your hamstring or shin, bringing it in closer to your chest, you will start to feel tension on the outside of your right hip. If you are unable to reach to your hamstring, it is a big sign that your hips are really tight.

These tests will make you understand your body's present ability of different motions around the major joints also and, also these tests can be performed with low intensity initially and, with time with regular monitoring the present conditions will improve and, you will be able to perform better with time and, that too without any injuries.

Different stretches will be discusses in the work out planning section.

CHAPTER 4

WORK OUT PRE REQUISITES AND, WORK OUT PLANNING

Work out pre-requisites

To start with, three biggest constraints that I have come across are

When to work out?

Where to work out?

What to work out?

Now when we have understood the present position of our body in terms of endurance, strength and, flexibility, it is also important to assess the resources we have or the infrastructure available for the work out.

Yes this phase is very important. Many of the people really want to do Body Transformation but are not able to either start or carry on much because they do not assess their resources well.

When to work out?

The biggest constraint I have seen is time

Yes its true, An office going person, a house wife, a college or school going student, a businessman, a government servant, People with irregular daily schedules who don't have time to work out at least. Here I will definitely say that we badly want to look good and, fit but it is not our priority. We always look for some shortcuts. I daily see articles, videos, blogs write-ups on how to get fit in minimum time and, minimum efforts and, we get attracted to it also.

In my fitness career of more than 30 years, I had to work out regularly and, watch my diet on constant basis. Apart from my competition days weight management in my daily routines had been a challenge. I have to work hard for it, definitely it was never a child's play. We have to keep our focus clear, if you want it then you have to make it your priority and, go to each and, every possible extent to achieve it. There were days when I used to be on business tours and, whole day I was in field, in those case I took membership of gyms on per day visit and, I used to make it sure to hit a gym, whether 5 in the morning or 10 at night and, if gym not possible I used to work out in my hotel room.

Yes, I agree its not easy and, there are no short cuts, as I have mentioned earlier that if we go for instant results, we will just lose some muscles and, water from our body and, nothing else. Fat have to be melted down by quality work outs and, balanced diet, trust me there is no other option. It is difficult but its not impossible, My book will not help you certainly, if you are looking for short cuts, yes it can be achieved faster by strict management but precisely no short cuts.

Consider the following points

1. Now talking about the time thing, let me assure you 20 minutes daily is enough for the start up. Yes you read it right. If you are doing your work outs at 60% to 80% of your intensity, trust me, any form of work out, whether it cardiovascular or strength or flexibility, any or mix of these, just 20 minutes is enough.

2. You can do your work outs in any part of the day, its not about doing it in the morning, afternoon or evening or at night, any time, just you have to take care of spacing your work outs from big meals. Just try and, understand, what is the basis behind a work out, one is to reach your target heart rate and, maintain it as long as possible, second is to initiate blood flow in each part of the body to strengthen it third is to increase the mobility around your joints,

that's it. Its no rocket science, you don't have to spend hours in the gym or have some grueling technically strong work outs given by highly qualified or certified gurus. Yes I agree the quality of the work out matters, u will definitely need a mentor, but nothing works if you don't do it. None of the lines or words in my book will work if you don't work out.

3. Its not necessary that you work out seven days a week, yes it is not necessary, just you need to schedule yourself. Also its not necessary that you have to touch all the aspects (cardio, strength, flexibility) in all your work outs. The first and, most important thing is to schedule your work outs. Generally people schedule their daily routine as per their work outs, and, make life complex, what happens is finally things get complex and, they have to stop their work outs out of frustration. Try and, schedule your work outs on the basis of your daily routines, find out a comfortable time, you can wake up 20 minutes early, or anytime throughout the day you can fix up your work outs. Also you can work out twice a week, as per the schedules and, cover all aspects. yes trust me, this works.

Time, is not the constraint, it's the will power and, determination that works

Where to work out?

Second issue we come across is infrastructure

The second most important concern which comes in picture is "Where to Work out".

Yes it does, It's a big question.

Now a days there are so many options, gyms, yoga centers, aerobic classes, parks, dancing, cycling, and, some new technical forms of fitness have come into picture like zumba, Pilates, MMA, ABT, Suspension training, Tai Chi and, many more But still no option. It's True.

We always get confused, when it comes to where to work out, as because of excess of knowledge around, we get fascinated towards some new and, more technical but complicated fundamentals. For those who have been doing work outs from long time, its good to challenge yourself with new things, but if you want to start a program stick to the basics. Never go for something that is really complex, and, you can not handle it after some time. If you want to learn or get specialized in a particular form of fitness then things are different.

When it come to Body Transformation, I really like to emphasise on the target oriented approach. We should be clear that what do we want from a particular work out.

Consider the following points.

1. First thing is Body adaptation. As per your body assessment done, in the previous chapters, figure out what you will be able to do and, maintain it for a period of time. Yes its really important. Imagine, someone having lower back issue and, he or she started power yoga or opted for high impact aerobic sessions, in that case we will end up increasing our pain and, get the condition worse, nothing else. Imagine someone with low bone density, opted for hardcore strength training, then he will find it really difficult to continue. Someone with medical complications like high blood pressure and, high cholesterol will not be able to sustain long work outs.

   So you must go for the option, which you can able to do it easily and, sustain for a period of time. Then gradually you increase the intensity or switch over to different forms of fitness.

2. Second aspect is access. Choose a work out place which is really accessible to you. Many a time I have seen people joining an institution or may be a fitness centre out of fascination and, excitement, but not able to continue because it's far off or timings are odd which doesn't suits you. It's really important, that the work out place should be in your reach, that will be easier for you to continue with your work outs.

3. People at the infrastructure matters a lot, the management, the faculty and, the peer group, it matters a lot. It's really important

to join a place, where you find likeminded and, motivated people, which helps you in carrying on with your work outs, as it is really important.

4. Join an institution, that is of your taste. If you personally like dance based fitness may be aerobics or zumba or something, then there is no point joining a yoga centre or a gym. You will not be able to be motivated by the people around and, also you will get bored very easily and, you will stop doing it.

What to work out?

Now the biggest question arises is what to do when it comes to work out??

What will be the best form of work out for Body Transformation?

Some says morning walk or jog is the best, some rely on gym, some insist on doing aerobics or dancing and, some says that only yoga is best for long time fitness results.

I will say it depends

Yes it depends on your body type, your internal body factors and, on your goals

Calculating your body type

Here, before starting the work out programming, the first thing you need to understand and, evaluate is your body type.

Depending on your Body Mass Index, Body Fat Percentage and, your hip waist ratio

We can divide the body type into three basic categories

Ectomorph - Lean and, Long, small delicate frame and, bone structure, hard to gain weight, lean muscle mass, fast metabolism.

Mesomorph – Athletic, generally hard body, well defined muscles, rectangular shaped body, strong, gain muscle easily, gain fat more easily than ectomorph

Endomorph – soft and, round body, gain muscle and, fat very easily, generally short, round physique, find it hard to lose fat, slow metabolism, muscle not so well defined.

These body types are not set in stone, In fact, most people have a combination of two body types. These combinations are either ectomorph/mesomorph or mesomorph/endomorph.

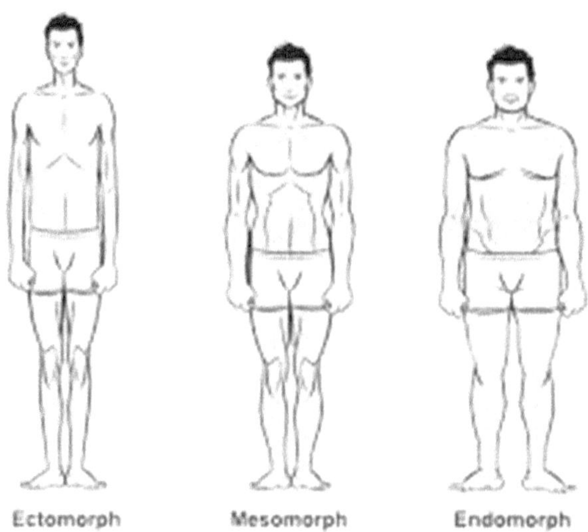

Body Types

Now the question comes how will you find out your body type

Step 1

Calculate your BMI as discussed in previous chapters

Step 2

Calculate your Hip waist ratio

Step 3

Get your fat percentage evaluated by a Body Composition Analysis machine

(If you are not able to get your body analysis done meanwhile, you can proceed with BMI and, Hip Waist ratio)

71

To describe the work out programming I am hereby giving some categories on the basis of which you may decide the work out you have to follow:

Category 1 – Ectomorph

BMI = 18 to 21

Males	Females
Waist hip ratio – up to 0.9	waist hip ratio – upto 0.8
Fat% - 6 to 9%	Fat % - 12-16

Category 2 – Ecto-mesomprph

BMI = 21 to 24

Males	Females
Waist hip ratio – 0.9 to 0.93	Waist hip ratio – 0.8 to 0.83
Fat% - 11 to 15%	Fat % - 17-21

Category 3 – Mesomorph

BMI = 24 to 27

Males	Females
Waist hip ratio – 0.93 to 0.96	Waist hip ratio – 0.83 to 0.86
Fat% - 16 to 20%	Fat % - 21 – 25%

Category 4 – Meso Endomorph

BMI = 27 to 30

Males	Females
Waist hip ratio – 0.96 to 0.99	Waist hip ratio – 0.86 to 0.89
Fat% - 20 to 25%	Fat % - 25 to 30%

Category 5 – Endomorph

BMI = above 30

Males	Females
Waist hip ratio – 1 or above	Waist hip ratio – 0.9 or above
Fat% - above 25	Fat % - above 30%

Here I would mention that, for people who have been into more of strength training from a long time, it is possible that there BMI will be on higher side, in that case I advise them to calculate their waist hip ratio and, get their body fat percentage checked by the body composition analysis machine and, relate all the data and, then only proceed with the given programmes.

Work out programming basics

As we have discussed when it comes to work outs, we have three different aspects

1. Cardiovascular Endurance
2. Strength Training
3. Flexibility

Now on the basis of our body type we have to decide the quantum of each aspect, lets discuss it category wise:

Category 1 – Ectomorph

BMI = 18 to 21

Males	Females
Waist hip ratio – up to 0.9	Waist hip ratio – upto 0.8
Fat% - 6 to 9%	Fat % - 12-16

Here as we can see the goal is to gain muscle weight, as the fat is already to a minimum level, In this category, strength based work out is more preferable that too with repetition count which lies between 6 to 8 repetitions per set. Endurance and, flexibility training can be done once or maximum twice a week. Compound training will be more preferable where more than one body part is involved at a given point of time and, also good rest between sets should be taken. Diet will also be a major criteria, calories should be in surplus. These category people will need good amount of energy in their work outs, pre work out, during work out and, post work out meals should be specially taken care of.

Category 2 – Ecto-Mesomprph

BMI = 21 to 24

Males	Females
Waist hip ratio – 0.9 to 0.93	Waist hip ratio – 0.8 to 0.83
Fat% - 11 to 15%	Fat % - 17-21

Here as we can see the goal is to gain muscle weight, but at the same time we need to take care of the increasing body fat also. In this category, strength based work out will be preferable but with repetition count which lies between 8 to 12 repetitions per set. Endurance and, flexibility training will be done two to three times a week. Compound training will be more preferable where more than one body part is involved at a given point of time but there will be less of rest between sets so that we can burn calories also. HIIT, high-intensity interval training should also be practiced and, cardio 20 to 30 minutes to extract out hidden fat.

No carbohydrates, only protein before cardio will definitely help.

Category 3 – Mesomorph

BMI = 24 to 27

Males	Females
Waist hip ratio – 0.93 to 0.96	Waist hip ratio – 0.83 to 0.86
Fat% - 16 to 20%	Fat % - 21 – 25%

Here as we can see, that it is more important to reduce the fat percentage as it is on the higher side, at the same time we have to preserve the muscle mass that is the good weight.

In this category the repetition count will lie between 12 to sixteen reps when comes to strength training.

Here I will recommend this person to take the endurance training seriously atleast three to four times daily and, that too for more than forty minutes.

This category, if not taken care will shift to endomorph really soon.

Category 4 – Meso Endomorph

BMI = 27 to 30

Males	Females
Waist hip ratio – 0.96 to 0.99	Waist hip ratio – 0.86 to 0.89
Fat% - 20 to 25%	Fat % - 25 to 30%

Here it is clearly visible that the fat percentage is high. WE should focus more on endurance and, flexibility training. As far as strength training is concerned it can be dome twice a week covering all the body part to maintain or develop the muscle mass.

Endurance and, flexibility training should be done four to five days a week and, in strength training also, the focus should be calorie burning, no rest training with supersets.

Category 5 – Endomorph

BMI = above 30

Males	Females
Waist hip ratio – 1 or above	Waist hip ratio – 0.9 or above
Fat% - above 25	Fat % - above 30%

This is the endomorph category, here the fat percentage has exceeded all the limits and, it is very much clear that this individual must be having metabolic syndrome. In that case most likely, chances of medical complications are also there like diabetes, thyroid malfunction, cholesterol issues blood pressure, stomach inflammation or any other. I would recommend that the medical aspects should also be taken care with work outs.

The endurance training will be primary in this case and, the person should try to initiate calorie difference in the body by consuming less food and, burning more calories.

Also strength training is important, so that the good weight increases and, the body metabolism increases which will increase the metabolism and, will help in improving the overall health.

How to design your work out

Now when we have understood our body type and, the basic plan of action, the biggest task is

What you have to do?

Here I will give you all the options from which you can select the exercises and, make a plan as per your body type, your strengths and, the limitations.

Let's start with endurance training first

Just try and, understand, what is endurance training, here the target is we have to achieve our heart rate and, maintain it for 20 to 40 minutes. Simple

So any activity that you can do it rhythmically in a nonstop pattern without dropping your heart rate.

1. Fast Walking to start with is the basics, We can jog or run also to achieve our heart beat and, maintain it for 20 to 40 minutes or above as per your capacity. You can do it outdoors or on a treadmill. You have to make sure that your heart rate is elevated otherwise you are waisting time. With time you can increase the speed and, gradually challenge your self in terms of speed, intensity and, time.

2. Cycling is also a good option, it can be outdoors or indoor.

3. An elliptical cross strainer is a good equipment you can use.

4. Activity based endurance training is also helpful like Aerobics, Dance, kick boxing or other group sessions or classes are really great to burn calories and, elevate your heart rate.

5. Self bodyweight exercises also, when done in a nonstop manner for more than twenty minutes without break elevates your heart rate and, at the same time increase your muscle strength also. This requires a lot of flexibility and, practice, when you will start practicing it, gradually you will get used to it. Here I will mention, self bodyweight training or the functional training or zero equipment training are really in practice but till you get accustomed to it or you are or you get perfect at it it will not be a good option. As first thing is you need strength to perform those, and, if you do not have muscle mass, in that case you will stop again and, again or take breaks or let me put it this way that the heart rate will be sky rocketed in seconds and, you will have to stop.

   So I strongly recommend, that depending on your goals and, body type you should opt for the endurance training options, where you can progressively elevate your heart rate and, maintain it for forty minutes and, above, remember its in rhythm and, non stop.

6. One point to mark here is, that your daily activities like people with hectic daily schedules and, especially housewife with household chores has this feeling that there daily routine is really hectic, so they do not have to work out, it's not so. I understand it is demanding and, is making you tired but when it come to work out basics they cannot be considered. As I have explained above, in endurance training it is really important to maintain the heart rate for 20 to 40 minutes, then only we get the desired results

   Self bodyweight exercises are mentioned in the strength section.

How to plan the flexibility training

Term flexibility as discussed earlier is the range of motion in a joint or series of joints, and, length in muscles that cross the joints to induce a bending movement or motion. It varies from person to person but it can be increased by exercise.

Fexibility training is not just some stretches, its more than that. I have seen flexibility is never taken seriously. Its not just 2 minutes in the beginning and, 2 minutes after the work out or when we just woke up we move our hands and, legs a bit.

Understanding all the joints and, the muscles we need to stretch and, I recommend proper session for the flexibility training atleast one or twice a week

To start with, we should start with all the flexibility tests mentioned in the flexibility chapter.

They are as follows:

1. Sit and, Reach

2. Toe Touch.

3. Groin stretch

4. Lateral side Bending

5. Trunk Rotation stretch

6. Shoulder Stretch

7. Hip Rotators stretch

All these exercises are to be done in one session.

Every stretch should be hold for 30 seconds each side and, should be done 3 to 5 times.

In every session you can choose five to seven stretches and, hold every stretch from 30 seconds to 1 minute and, do it three to five times. This should be practiced two to three times a week depending on r your body type, fat percentage and, fitness goals.

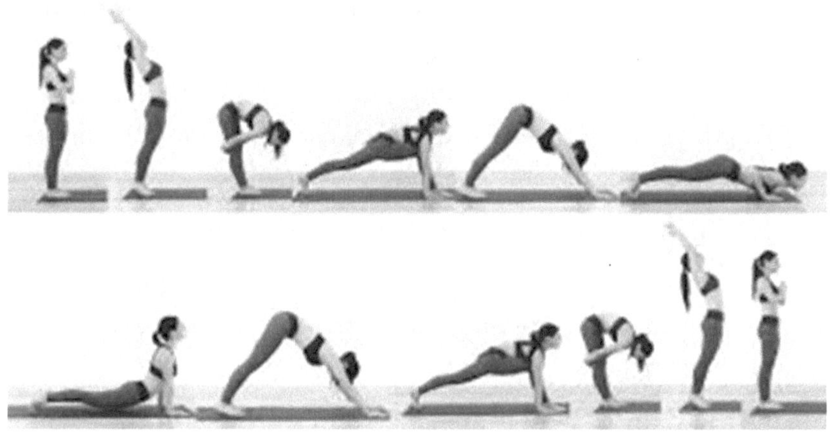

Suryanamaskar

Suryanamaskar - or the Sun Salutation, is a practice in yoga as exercise incorporating a sequence of some twelve gracefully linked asana or body positions. The basic sequence involves moving from a standing position into downward and, upward dog poses and, then back to the standing position, but many variations are possible.

I personally recommend doing suryanamaskar in your exercise program, in addition to maintaining cardiovascular health and, muscle activation it helps in stretching

You can start with rounds of suryanamaskar and, gradually increase it as per your capacity and, goals.

How to plan the strength training with equipment or without equipments

I Hereby divide strength training into five sections

Push Movements

Pull Movements

Lateral movements

Core training (abdominals and, lower back)

Lower Body Exercises

1. Push Movements Exercises – A push exercise is performed when the muscle pushes the weight away from the body during the concentric or the contracting phase of the movement and, then lengthens in the eccentric or the extending phase when the weight is moved back towards the body

Un Equipped Training or without any equipment

1. Pushups – Normal grip, close grip, wide grip, inclined or decline push-ups and, other variations also (please see the pics shown here)

   Pushup is a good exercise, you can do it, it is a compound exercise and, it targets our chest, shoulder, triceps, back, core and, lower body also to some extend.

2. Reverse Dips or Dips behind the back -- Grip Wide, shoulder width or close grip

It is a good exercise for the shoulders, triceps and, chest also. The intensity can be varied by the position of the legs.

Equipped Training or with the equipment (with dumbbells, barbell, weights and, bench)

All the exercises can be done at home also with minor equipments at place or if you don't want to invest in equipments you can take a strength rope also. It all depends on your goals

1. Bench Press for chest, shoulder and, triceps primarily all the grips and, with dumbbell or barbell

2. Inclines Bench Press for upper chest, shoulders and, triceps, same as above

3. Shoulder Presses for all the heads of the shoulders, same as above

4. Parallel Bar Dips

5. Tricep push downs

6. Lying, standing, or seated tricep extensions with dumbbells or barbell

2. Pull Movements Exercises – A pull exercise on the other hand, is performed when the muscle pulls weight toward the body during the concentric or contracting portion of the movement and, then lengthens as the weight moves away from the body during the eccentric or extending portion when the weight is moved back from the body.

Un Equipped training or without any equipment

1. Chin ups or pull ups – any grip

2. Inverted Rows

Equipped Training or with the equipment (with dumbbells, barbells, weights, or strength ropes

1. Lat pull downs – all grips

2. Rowing movements, seated or standing with cables, Barbells, dumbbells

3. Bicep Curls standing or seated with dumbbells or barbells or cable

3. Lateral Movements for upper body – The lateral raises with barbells or dumbbells can be done either ways to the side, front or rear of the body. These are certain isolation exercises for upper body muscle development. They can be done empty handed, with strength ropes or dumbbells and, barbells.

4. Core strengthening exercises – Core exercises are an important part of a well rounded fitness program. Aside from the occasional sit ups and, certain leg raises, however, core exercises are often neglected. Core exercises train the muscles in your pelvis, lower back, hips and, abdomen to work in harmony. This leads to better balance and, stability, whether in sports or daily activities. In fact, most of the physical activities depend on the stable core muscles.

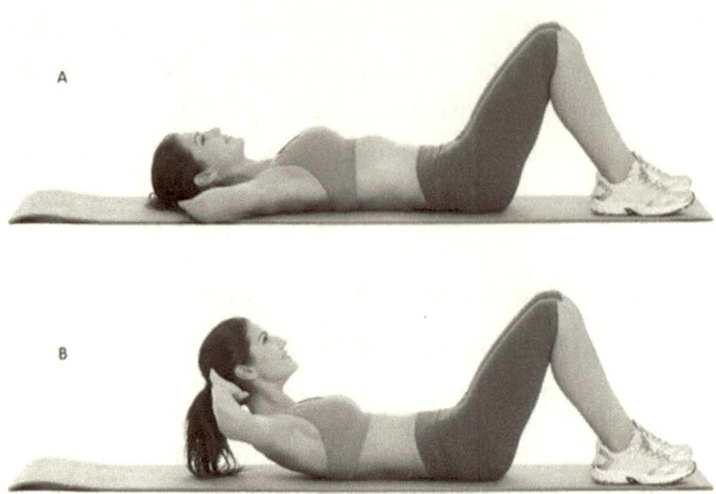

Crunches

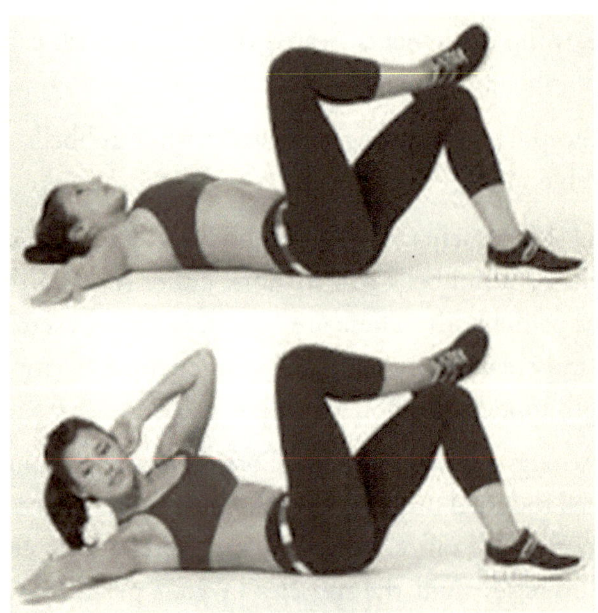

Oblique Crunches

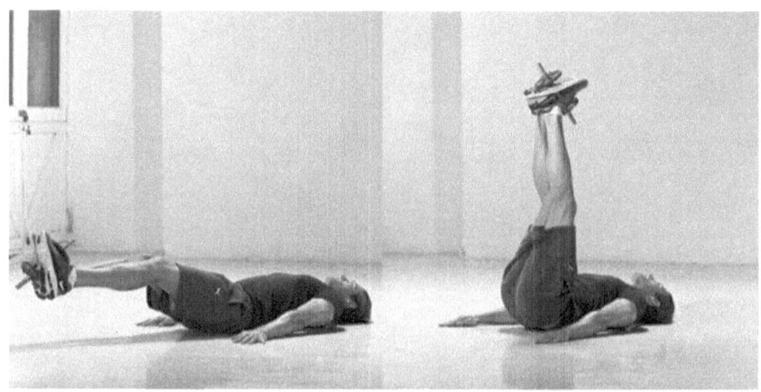

leg-raise

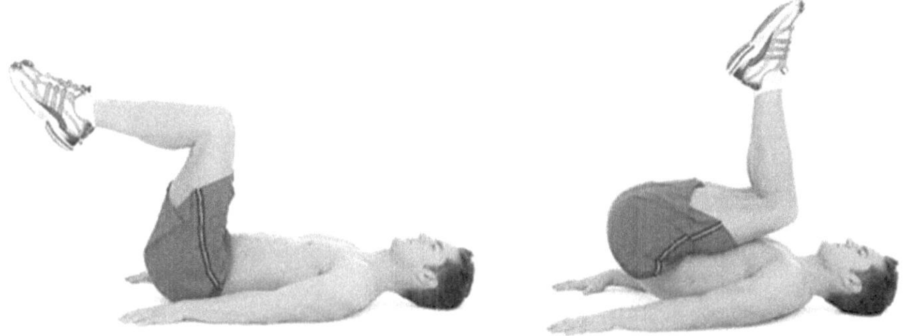

Reverse Crunches

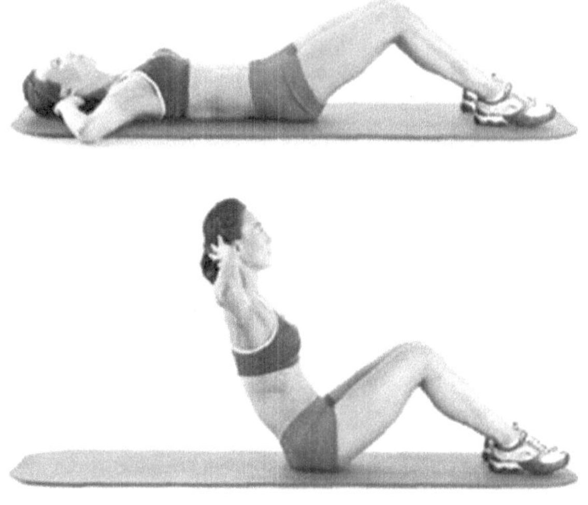

Sit ups

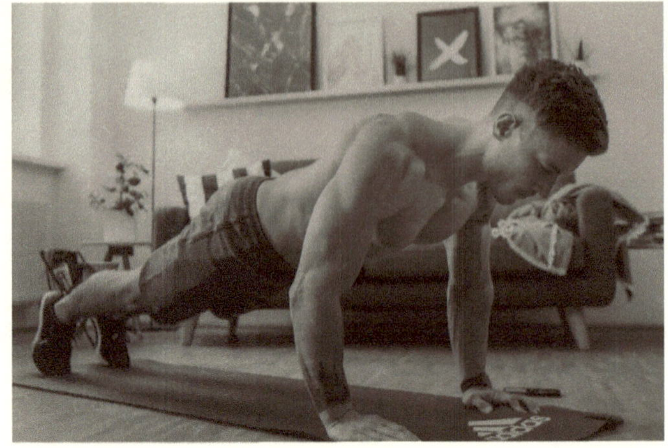

Plank

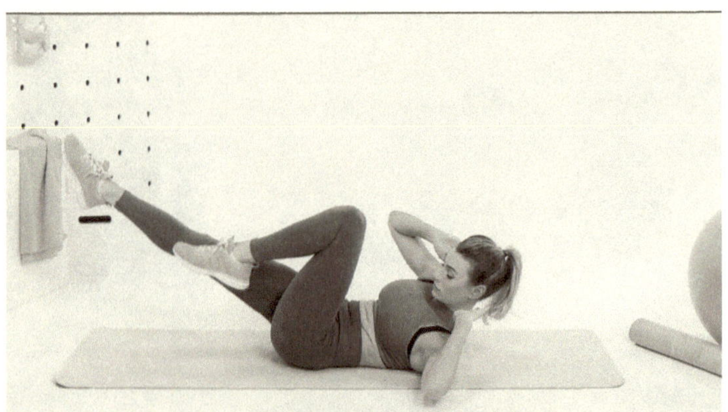

Cycling Crunches

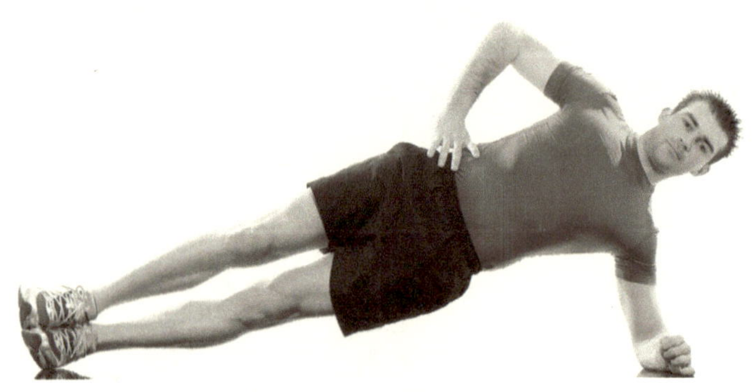

Side plank

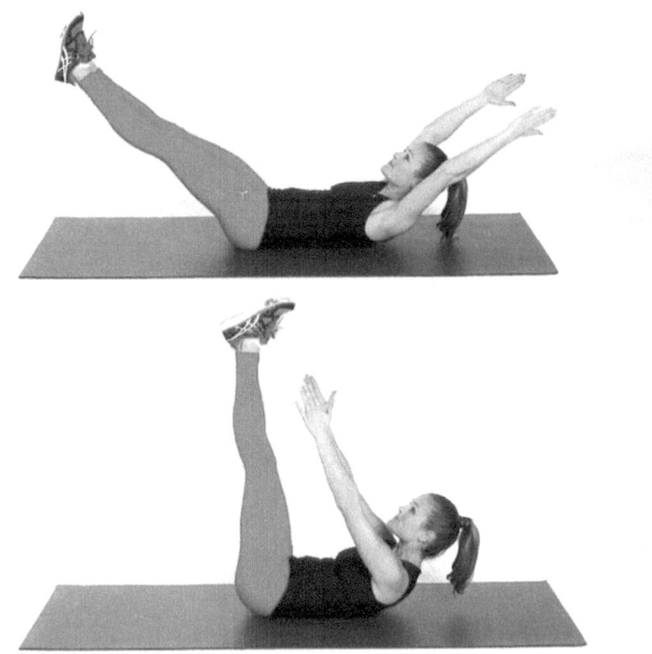

Compound crunches

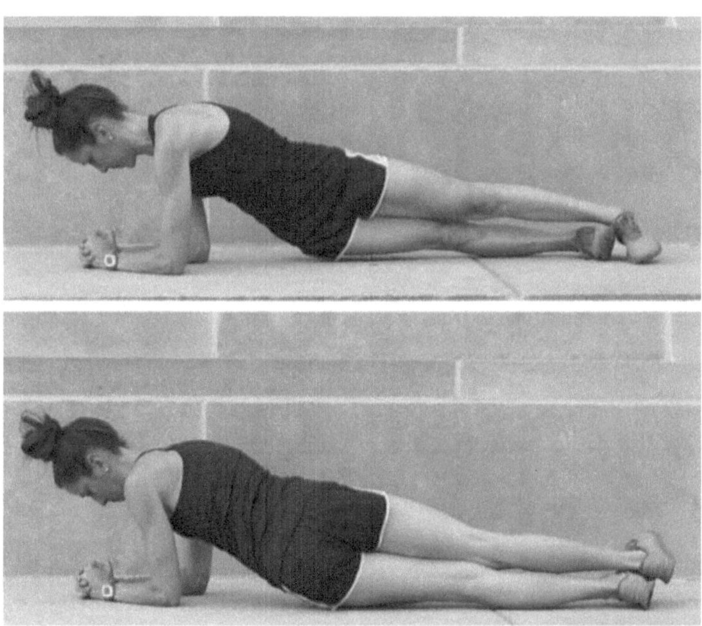

Plank Twist

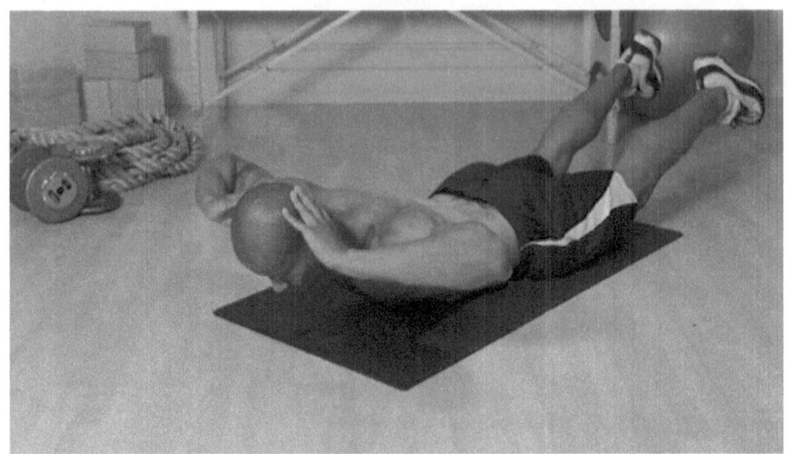

Hyper extension

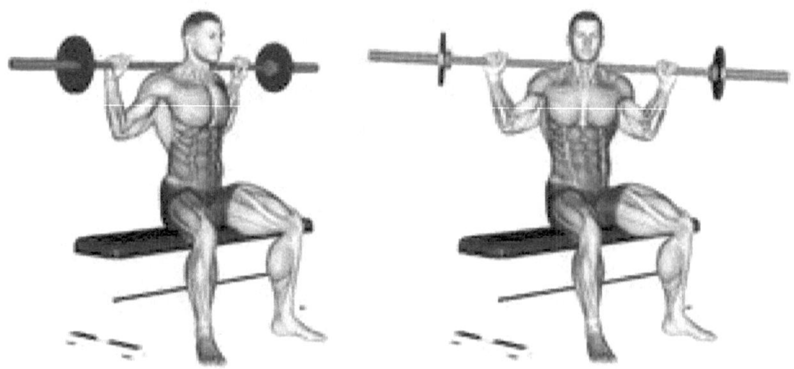

Seated Twist

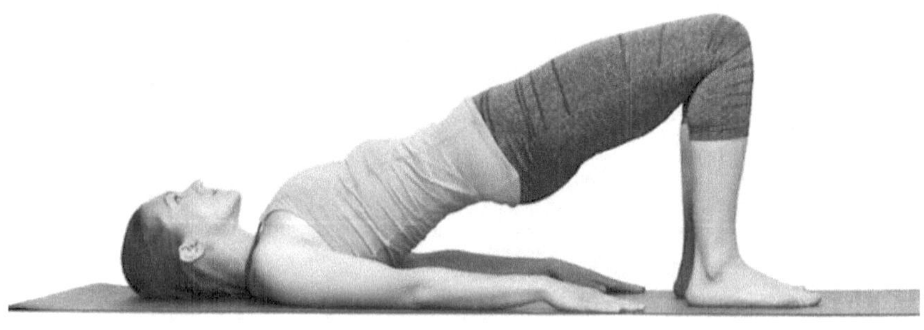

Glute-Bridge

a. Crunches

b. Oblique crunches

c. Flat or inclined leg raises

d. Reverse Crunches

e. Sit ups

f. Planks – full or elbow

g. Cycling crunches

h. Side planks

i. Compound Crunches

j. Plank twist

k. Hyper Extensions

l. Side Bends

m. Seated Side twists

n. Glute Bridges

5. Lower body Exercises – It probably comes no surprise that having strong legs can take you far. Even if you are not training for a race or working toward any other specific athletic goal, you need legs that are strong enough to literally carry you through life. Everything from walking up a flight of stairs to lifting your heavy laundry bag is easier when you can put some leg muscle behind it. The main objective is to train all the segments – Quads, Hamstrings, Glutes and, calves

Un Equipped or Without any Equipments

Luckily, effective leg exercises don't have to be complicated and, they can be done at home also. There are plenty of bodyweight leg exercises you can add to your work out routine to get stronger and, work toward any bigger strength and, performance goals you may have too.

Exercises are as follows

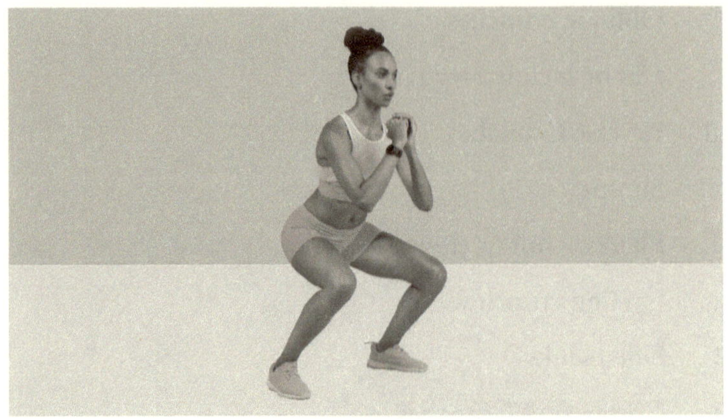

Squats

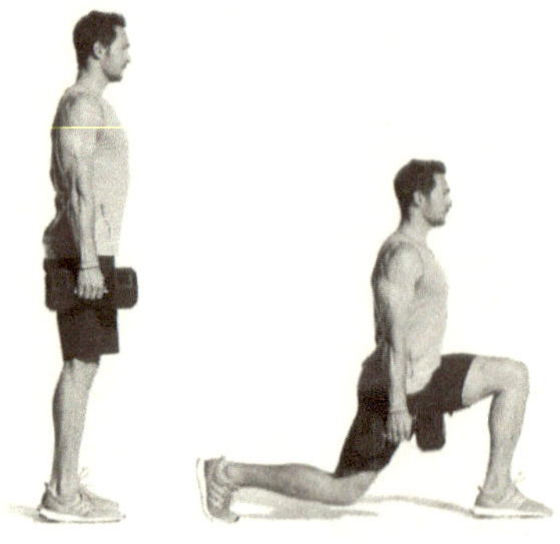

Lunges

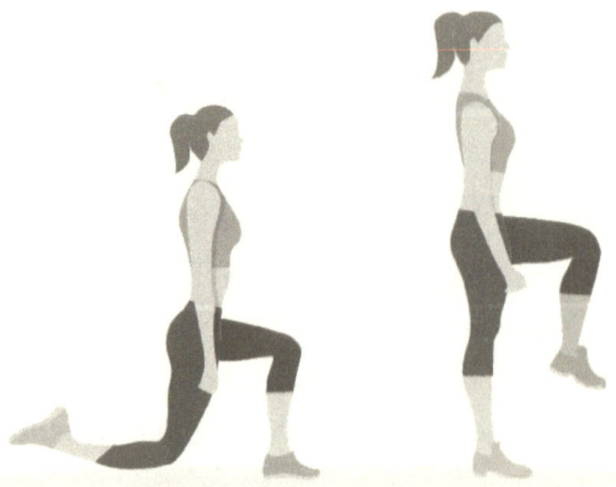

Reverse lunge with Knee Lift

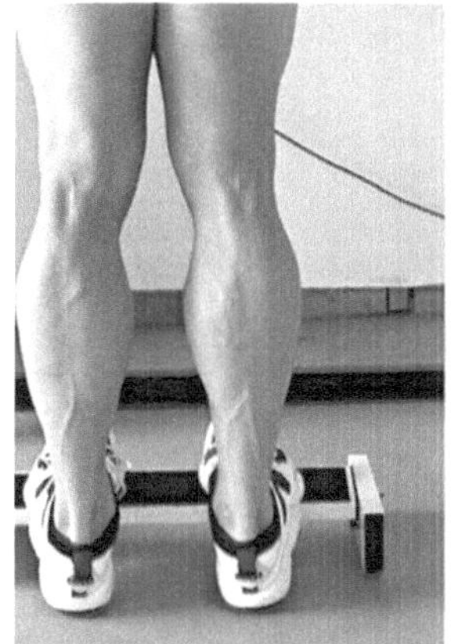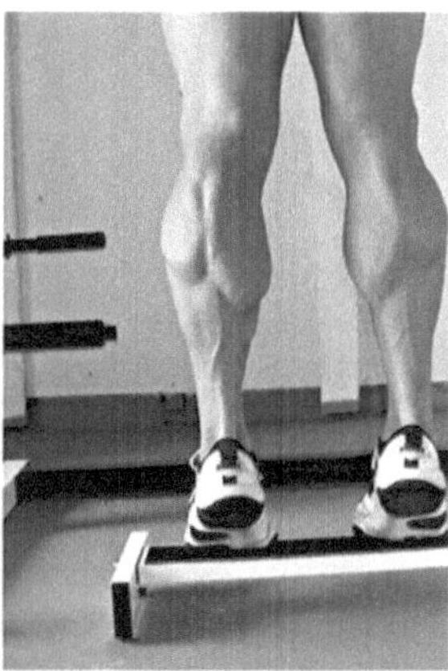

Calf Raises

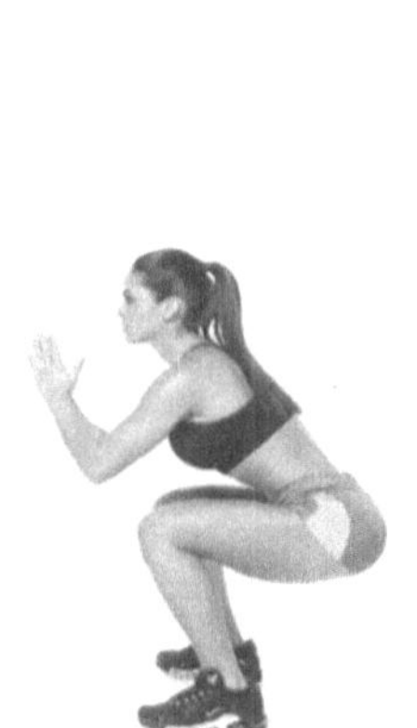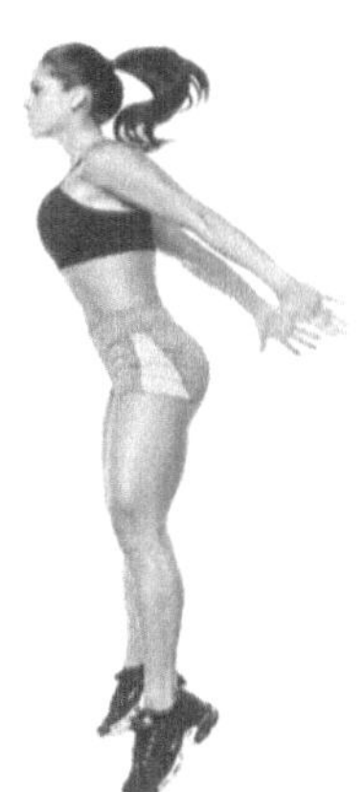

Jump-squat

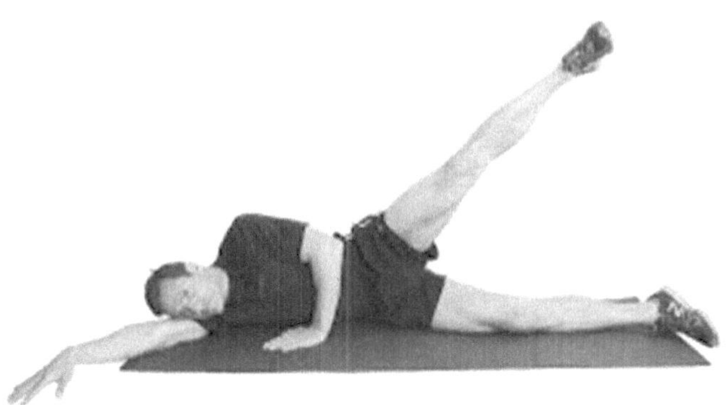

Side leg lift

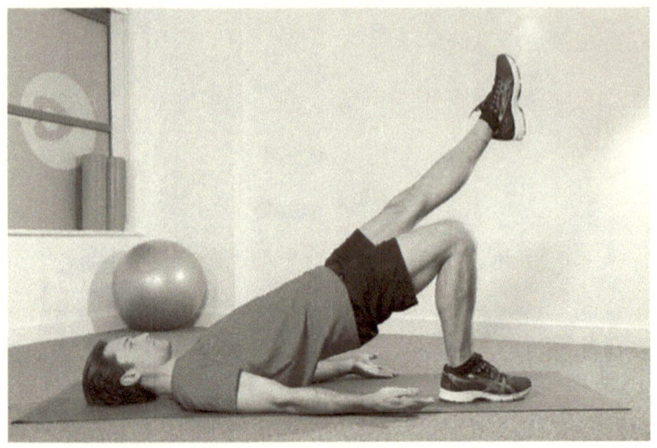

Glute bridge variation

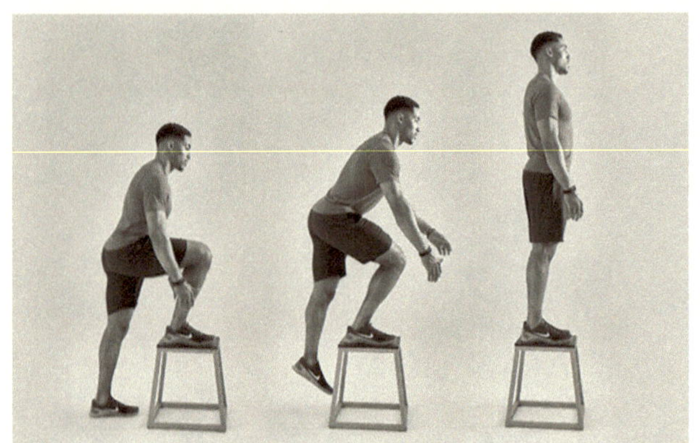

Box step ups

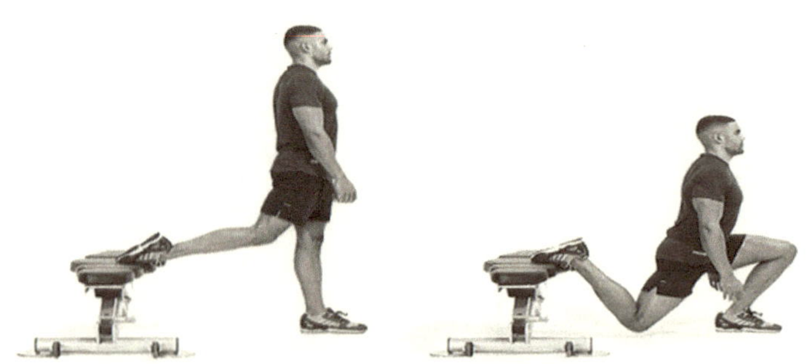

BULGARIAN SPLIT SQUAT

Bulgarian-Split-Squat

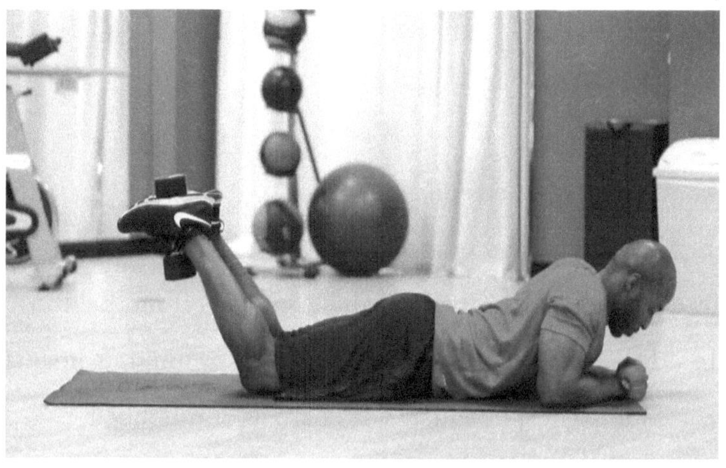

Lying leg curls

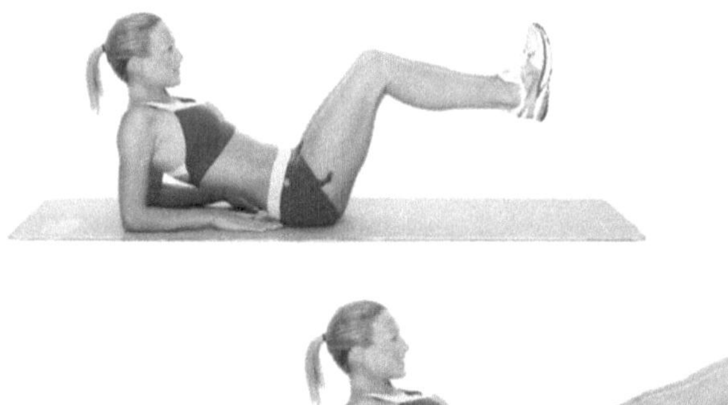

Lying leg extensions

a. Squats – close, shoulder width, wide leg, pistol

b. Lunges – forward, reverse and, towards sides and, back cross

c. Reverse lunge with knee lifts

d. Calf raises

e. Squat jumps

f. Lying side leg raises, upper leg and, lower leg

g. Glute bridges, all types

h.   Box step ups

i.   Bulgarian split squats

j.   Lying leg curls

k.   Lying leg extensions

Equipped or with Equipments

a.   Barbell or Dumbell weighted squats – front, behind

b.   Deadlifts – conventional, straight leg, sumo, Romanian

c.   Bulgarian split squats with barbell or dumbbell

d.   Glute Ham raise

e.   Leg curls

f.   Leg extensions

g.   Weighted glute bridges

h.   Lunges with barbell or dumbbell – stationary, forward reverse or walking

Now we have understood all the basics of training and, their exercises as under

Endurance training and, exercises

Flexibility training and, exercises

Strength training and, exercises

Importance of self bodyweight exercises

In all the above discussion I have mentioned the un equipped or exercises without any equipment or precisely I must say *self bodyweight exercises.*

If practiced properly and, regularly in a specialized manner, Bodyweight exercises are all you need to build a lean and, mean machine. Thankfully, carving a great physique does not take a bench, a barbell, an equipment or a dumbbell, all it takes is you. Yes, am serious.

Bodyweight exercises are not only time savers, they are extremely effective also. A study published in the American college of sports medicine's Health and, fitness journal found that bodyweight exercises are an efficient way to decrease body fat, and, boost muscular fitness.

In today's world, people are not able to give time for work outs, these type of program can offer a good option to help busy individuals improve their health and, at the time manage their stress levels also.

Self bodyweight exercises are really accessible, increase mobility and, stability, develop technique, prevent injuries, are quick and, easy and, most important is you can emphasize on all the aspects endurance, strength and, flexibility at the same time. Also I will mention that if done correctly you can burn good calories faster than any other program.

Some of the exercises are

Pushups, pull ups, Planks, Walk forward with hands and, walk back, Glute bridges, inverted rows, mount climbers, burpee, Dips, squats, split squats, Back extensions, Box jumps, side planks, plank to pushups, plank marches, clap pushups, spider man pushups, bicycle crunches, handstand pushups and, many more

CHAPTER 5

MEAL PLANNING

It really took me two days to write the first line of this chapter, yes it id

"Food is your friend, and, not your enemy", none of the world's best work outs can help you if you think that food will make you fat, If you are really serious about Body Transformation, make this clear in your mind.

but yes the following questions need to be seriously taken care:

Why to eat?

How much to eat?

When to eat?

What to eat?

Yes, all the above questions need to be answered and, that too precisely and, nail on the head

Let's start with why to eat

Whenever you decide you have to get fit, what is the first thing you do?

We start cutting down on our diet.

Yes we do, calorie restricted diet is the most common approach when it comes to Fitness, but the most dangerous thing which could kick start lot many problems inside your body.

Before answering this question We need to understand what is body metabolism because one of the main reasons that losing weight is so difficult with calorie restricted diets is because of the impact that it has on your metabolism.

Understanding the body metabolism

Metabolism is the term for a set of chemical reactions that occur in the cells of living organisms to sustain life. The metabolic process lead to growth and, reproduction and, allow living organisms to maintain their structures and, respond to the surrounding environment. All chemical reactions, from digestion to transport of substances from cell to cell, are part of metabolism.

Metabolism Influences your basic energy needs, how much you intake with how much physical activity you get are the things that ultimately determine your weight.

Metabolism is the process by which your body converts food into energy. During this complex biochemical process, calories are combined with oxygen to release the energy your body needs to function.

Even when you are at rest, I repeat even when you are rest, your body needs energy for all its internal – known and, unknown functions like breathing, blood circulation, hormonal level adjustments, growing repairing cells, digestion and, many more.

The number of calories your body uses to carry out all these basic functions is known as basal metabolic rate, what you might call metabolism.

Basic factors affecting metabolism:

a. Your body size and, composition – people with more muscle mass, burn more calories, even at rest

b. Men usually have less minimum body fat requirements than women of the same age and, weight, their basal metabolic rate is high

c. As you get older, muscle mass decreases if we don't work out, slowing down calorie burning

Here I will mention that In addition to basal metabolic rate, two other factors determine how many calories your body burns each day:

a. Food Processing or Thermogenesis – Digesting, absorbing, transporting and, storing the food you consume also takes calories. About 10 % of the calories from carbohydrates and, protein you eat are used during the digestion and, absorption of the food and, nutrients.

b. Physical Activity:

It can be divided into two parts

1. Non-exercise activity Thermogenesis - this activity includes daily home or house activities, or in proper terms I will say, an activity where we nor reach our heart rate and, if in case we reach it we are not able to maintain it due to short duration of the activity. Like catching a bus, or climbing a stair etc

2. Exercise activity Thermogenesis – this activity includes proper work out routine where target heart rate is achieved and, maintained also for 20 to 40 minutes. Jogging, playing a sport or swimming etc.

Effects of fasting and, crash diet

Now coming back to our question

Why to eat?

Let's see what happens when we cut our calories for prolonged period

Before explaining it technically, what happens when you restrict your diet, I would give an example

As am writing this book in the crucial covid – 19, lock down period, I will take its example.

In the lock down period everything is locked up, none of the shops are open, only the necessities are available, that too in very limited quantities.

In this case what is happening, what we are doing is consuming really less resources, take it as food, and, also we are trying to store food in what ever form we can for future use. Because we do not know what policies are coming next, and, whether will we be able to get the necessities or not. In simple words we have lost the trust on the external environment, simply we are in a SOS mode that is save our souls.

Same happens, when cut down our calories, surprised right, yes it does

Our basal metabolic rate, is the minimum calories we require to maintain all the necessary chemical reactions inside the body, as discussed above, now when we restrict our calories for prolonged period following things happen

1. Body decreases the energy expenditure overall, as we reduce the consumption of the food in the lock down period, body senses a state of emergency or lock down.. In this case body reduces the calories expended in different forms like

   Resting energy expenditure - metabolism

   Non resting energy expenditure that is Non-exercise activity thermo genesis

   Thermogenic effect of food – burning of food

   Exercise activity Thermogenesis that is calories expended while work out

   That is the standard calorie expenditure is reduced

2. Body start storing the energy in forms of high calorie food that is fat, like in lock down period we start storing the foods for future use. Like we lost the trust on the external environment, your body lose trust in you and, start storing calories. Here I ll mention 1 gram of carbohydrates and, protein each is 4 calories and, 1 gram of fats is 9 calories and, its dense too, so body stores calories in form of fat.

In this manner you can see that reducing calorie intake or fasting for prolonged period never works.

In addition to cutting down calories a general approach or methodology to reduce fat is to increase the work outs. You plan it as a double attack, one is to reduce the calories and, second is to burn more calories in order to achieve your target faster.

Now is the time to understand this mechanism technically, How this planned double attack fails drastically.

Explanation 1

Whenever we reduce our energy intake, two things happen. One is energy deficit or the calorie deficit second is our body mass index (fat mass plus muscle mass) goes down. This signals the body for metabolic adaptation that means, your body alters the number of calories that it burns in necessary bio chemical reactions, in an attempt to preserve muscle mass. This is primarily achieved through a reduction in TRH and, TSH – these are the circulating thyroid hormones, also reducing the mitochondrial efficiency that is the cell to cell transfer of nutrients and, many other, collectively discussed above as metabolism. These changes are known as starvation mode or the metabolic adaptation.

In this case the resting energy expenditure is reduced nearly by 30%, that means if a person whose basic needs is 2000 calories reduces on prolonged basis, in that case 600 calories are less expended by the body.

Explanation 2

The calories expended by the body has a natural phenomenon, as written below

1. Resting energy expenditure - metabolism accounts for 70% of the energy expenditure.

2. Non Resting energy expenditure – Non-exercise activity Thermogenesis – accounts for the 15% of the energy expenditure.

3. Thermogenic effect of food accounts for the 10% energy expenditure

4. Only 5% of the of the calories are effectively expended by exercise activity thermo genesis.

    The total makes it 100%

Here, we get to understand two things

a. If we cut down calorie intake, body achieves a state of metabolic adaptation, reduces its resting energy expenditure, that is metabolism to nearly 40%, that shows for a 2000 calories diet, it reduces 600 less calories on daily basis, that was actually free or effort less for you.

b. Second is, only 5% of the calories are expended by the work out we do. That means if we increase our work out from 1 hour to 2 hours, earlier we were expending 100 calories, now we will be expending actually 200 calories which will be effectively helping us in losing fat.

So in order to create a calorie deficit, we ate less, work out more, but the effective result was of no use.

That is why in 99% of these practices we never lose fat or the lost weight comes back as we get back to our normal diet.

Metabolic Syndrome and, its effects

Here I would like to mention a word Metabolic Syndrome

Metabolic Syndrome describes a group of traits and, habits that raise the risk for coronary heart diseases, diabetes and, stroke. Risk factors include excess fat in the stomach, a high triglyceride level, low level of good cholesterol, high blood pressure and, high fasting blood sugar. These factor commonly occur together. This shows that when metabolism gets low it leads to further complications also.

It is becoming increasingly common as a result of the rise in obesity rates.

As we can see due to prolonged fasting it not only becomes difficult to lose fat but also many health problems start which leads to medical complications.

This shows Why you have to eat a healthy and, balanced eat.

Difference between water loss / muscle loss and, actual fat loss

There are many popular diets now a days which promises immediate results like lose 5 kg in a week or 10 to 20 kg in a month.

1 gram fat = 9 calories

1 kg of fat = 9000 calories

Logically we need to burn approximately 3500 calories to burn one pound of fat or burn 7000 calories to burn 1 kg of fat.

Now to proceed further, if we create a 500 calorie deficit on daily basis, in seven days we will be able to burn half kg of fat, 14 days – 1kg of fat and, finally approx a month to burn 2 kg of fat ideally.

So how on earth is possible to burn 10 kg of fat in one month, any diet or any fitness regime, will not be able to do this (excluding, certain extreme cases which are only viable for fitness professionals and, athletes for special short term goals like stage competitions).

Here I would mention that yes it is possible to lose 10 kg weight but its really difficult to lose 10 kg of fat. But I admit that I have seen people losing 10 kg of weight. Now what is that?

As we have discussed earlier Body has two mass – fat mass and, fat free mass or the muscle mass

Now coming to the special diets

In all these diet, they generally exclude carbohydrates in all forms and, salt, increase the quantity of salads and, tea or coffee.

The primary source of food is fats and, proteins.

One thing you have to remember that Carbohydrates and, salt, hold water inside the body, In this case what happens is due to the absence of carbohydrates and, water, body is not able to hold its water content and, we excrete a lot of water. Consequently the bodyweight comes down remember not fat but bodyweight.

The second mechanism which takes place in these diet is the action of the diuretics.

Any kind of tea or coffee helps in excreting out water from the body, so the excess use of tea and, coffee also helps to lose further water hence bodyweight comes down.

Also the use of salads or fruits, which increases urination also does the same job, water loss and, hence weight loss.

So the entire strategy focuses on excreting out maximum water from the body, which results in muscle loss also and, the weighing scale makes you happy by showing some reduced figures.

This is not fat loss, its just muscle and, water loss, and, trust me its not permanent, there will be a point when the body will not drain further water, and, you will be pale, weak and, having lost all the essential nutrients of the body, you will be having many medical complications.

One thing I would mention here is that carbohydrates also prevent protein from being used as an energy source, and, when we stop the intake of carbohydrates muscle loss is bound to happen.

Also the moment you will shift to normal diet, or the healthy diet you will gain all the weight again.

So do not get fascinated about some catchy or cheesy lines like "lose 10 or 20 kg in a month "

The above facts prove that you have to eat the minimum or the calculated amount of calories (given below) to have long lasting results.

Remember we have to get fit and, then look fit, not just look fit for some time.

How much to eat?

Calculating the total calories required

Before starting anything, we need to know our total calories intake as per our goals.

Formulae for calculating how much calories you need to eat

Step 1

For Females

(Weight in pounds x 4.35) + (height in inches x 4.7) – (agex4.7) + 655 = Basal metabolic rate

For Males

(Weight in pounds x 6.23) +(height in inches x 12.7) – (age x 6.8) + 66 = Basal metabolic rate

Step 2

Multiply it with the daily activity level factor

Life style – sedentary with work out 1-2 days a week - Multiply BMR by 1.2

Life style – moderately active with work out 2-3 days a week - Multiply BMR by 1.375

Life style Active with work out 3 to 5 days a week - Multiply BMR by 1.55

Life style super active with work out 5-6 days a week – Multiply by 1.725

Step 3

The calories calculated in step 2 are the calories required to maintain your bodyweight.

If the target is fat loss then subtract it by 500

Now the final product comes which you need to take for fat loss

That is known as the 500 calories deficit a day which is a healthy way to lose fat.

Here I will give you a simpler formulae for calculating the minimum calories you require on daily basis to lose fat in a healthy manner without disturbing your metabolism and, internal hormonal factors

Minimum calories you should take, when you are aiming for fat loss – bodyweight in kg x 2.2 x (10)

For highly active people and, people with good muscle count – the formulae will be

Bodyweight x 2.2 x 12

This will give you the amount of calories you have to take to lose fat effectively.

(I have explained this below with an example)

Now coming to the distribution of these calories

What are proteins and, calculating the amount of protein intake

1. Protein –

    To maintain and, develop the muscle count inside the body

    The amount of protein required on daily basis varies from 0.8 gram per kg of bodyweight to 1.2 gram per kg of bodyweight depending on the body composition, daily routine, type of work out and, the desired goals. Her I would mention that in case of professional athletes and, body builders, the demand of protein may go upto 2 gram per kg of bodyweight also.

    Like a girl weighing 60 kg and, height 5feet 3 inches may take 48 to 60grams of protein daily to maintain her muscle mass.

Food	Protein Rating
Eggs (whole)	100
Fish	70
Lean beef	69
Cow's milk	60
Brown rice	57
White rice	56
Soybeans	47
Whole-grain wheat	44
Peanuts	43
Dry beans	34
White potato	34

Food	% Protein by Weight	% Net Protein Utilization
Eggs	12	94
Milk	4	82
Fish	18–25	80
Cheese	22–36	70
Brown rice	8	70
Meat and fowl	19–31	68
Soybean flour	42	61

(Whey, a milk derivative, which is a refined product, has even more net protein than eggs.)

Essence of fats and, their daily intake

2. Fat –

    Dietary fats are essential to give your body energy, support cell growth, help protect your organs and, keep body warm. Fat also help absorb some nutrients and, produce important hormones too.

    Fat tends to be considered "bad" because it is associated with weight gain and, high cholesterol. However certain types of fat in appropriate proportions are important to be consumed. The key is to understand how to choose the right amount of each type of fat.

    The total dietary reference intake of fat in adults is 20% to 30% fat

    Fats can be further categorized as –

    a. Unsaturated fats – These fats are usually liquid at room temperature, sources include monounsaturated and, polyunsaturated fats. These fats help in lowering the bad cholesterol levels and, should be consumed in place of saturated fats. These are of two types –

        Monounsaturated fat - 10% to 15% - (olive, canola, peanut oils, nuts and, nut butters, olives and, avocado)

        Poly unsaturated fat – 5% to 10% (safflower, sunflower, corn, soybean, cottonseed oils, nuts. Omega 3 are a type of polyunsaturated fats which have heart protective benefits and, lower inflammation. Salmon, tuna, flaxseeds, chia seeds and, walnuts have omega 3.

    b. Saturated fat – less than 10% These are generally solid or waxy at room temperature and, mostly from animal sources. Taking too much of these is linked with raising bad cholesterol levels in blood and, increase internal inflammation. Example – beef, pork, lamb, skin of poultry, high fat dairy products, butter, tropical oils like palm and, coconut, baked goods like cookies and, pastries. People who are looking forward to body transformation, these fats are big no.

    c. Trans fat – 0%. These fatty acids are formed when a liquid fat is changed into solid fat through a process of hydrogenation. Many manufacturers use hydrogenated oils as an ingredient because it extends the shelf life and, the consistency of the foods. These fats decrease good cholesterol and, increase bad cholesterol. There are no safe levels for these, please avoid them completely.

d. Cholesterol – less than 300 mg per day. Cholesterol is made by the liver. Therefore, only animal based foods contain cholesterol. If your cholesterol levels are normal, limit the intake upto 300mg per day. If it is high limit the intake up to 200mg per day.

	Calories	Carbohydrate (gm)	Fat (gm)
Grain Group			
Bagel	163	31	1
Whole wheat bread, 1 slice	61	11	1
White bread, 1 slice	64	12	1
French bread, 1 slice	81	15	1
Bread sticks, 2	77	15	1
Graham crackers, 2 squares	60	11	1
Saltines, 10	125	20	4
Oatmeal, Quaker, ¾ cup	105	18	2
English muffin	135	26	1
Life Cereal, Quaker, ⅔ cup	111	19	2
Pancake, 4-inch dia.	61	9	2
Pasta, ½ cup	100	19	1
Rice, ½ cup	112	25	0
Flour tortilla, 8-inch dia.	105	18	3

Carbohydrates and, their daily intake

3. Carbohydrates – They provide fuel for the central nervous system and, energy for working muscles. They also prevent protein from being used as an energy source and, enable fat metabolism.

The number of carbohydrates a person should eat every day for weight loss varies depending on their age, sex, body type and, activity levels. The dietary guidelines recommends that Carbohydrates should consist of 45 to 65% of your total calorie count.

They are classified as simple or complex. The difference between the two forms is the chemical structure and, how quickly the sugar is absorbed and, digested. Simple carbs are digested and, absorbed more quickly and, easily than complex carbs.

Carbohydrates are good and, bad.

Bad carbs include pastries, sodas, highly processed foods and, white flour foods.

Good carbs are whole grains, fruits, vegetables, beans and, legumes, These carbs not only processes more slowly, but they also contain a lot of nutrients.

	Calories	Carbohydrate (gm)	Fat (gm)
Milk Group			
2% milk, 1 cup	121	12	5
Skim milk, 1 cup	86	12	0
Lowfat yogurt, 1 cup	225	42	3
Cottage cheese, 1 cup	164	7	2
Lowfat cheddar cheese	80	8	5
Lowfat American cheese	72	6	4
Lowfat mozzarella cheese	79	8	5
Meat Group			
Lean ground beef, 3 oz.	214	0	14
Flank steak, 3 oz.	209	0	12
Chicken, light meat w/o skin, roasted, 3 oz.	148	0	4
Chicken, dark meat, w/o skin, roasted, 3 oz.	176	0	8
Turkey, light meat, w/o skin, roasted, 3 oz.	135	0	3
Turkey, dark meat, w/o skin, roasted, 3 oz.	160	0	6
Turkey sandwich slices, 1 oz.	44	0	1
Tuna, spring water, 1 oz.	60	0	1
Rainbow trout, broiled, 3 oz	129	0	4
Salmon, 3 oz.	99	0	3
Beans, refried, 1 cup	270	47	3
Kidney beans, 1 cup	216	40	1
Ham, lean, 3 oz.	124	1	5
Peas, black-eyed, 1 cup	198	36	1
Peanut butter, 1 Tbsp.	95	2	8

	Calories	Carbohydrate (gm)	Fat (gm)
Fruits			
Apple, medium	80	20	0
Applesauce, ½ cup	53	14	0
Apricots, dried, 4 halves	33	9	0
Banana, medium	105	27	0
Cantaloupe, 1 cup pieces	57	13	0
Cherries, sweet, 10	49	11	0
Dates, dried, 10	228	61	0
Grapefruit, 1 half	39	10	0
Grapes, 1 cup	58	16	0
Orange	65	16	0
Peach	37	10	0
Pear	98	25	0
Pineapple, 1 cup pieces	77	19	0
Raisins, ¼ cup	300	79	0
Strawberries, 1 cup	45	11	0
Watermelon, 1 cup	50	12	0
Vegetables			
Asparagus, 6 spears	22	4	0
Green beans, ½ cup	22	5	0
Broccoli, ½ cup	23	4	0
Carrots, 1 medium	31	7	0
Cauliflower, ½ cup	15	3	0
Celery, 1 stalk	6	2	0
Corn, ¼ cup	89	21	0
Green peas, ¼ cup	67	13	0
Baked potato	220	51	0
Mushrooms, ½ cup	9	2	0
Spinach, ¼ cup	6	1	0
Tomato	24	6	0

Understanding the glycemic index and, glycemic index of different foods

A number of different types of carbohydrates have been studied, using white bread as the standard, to determine which might be optimal for glycogen re synthesis. White bread is assigned a glycemic index

GI of 100. Carbohydrates that quickly emptied into the blood stream (high glycemic) are recommended immediately after exercise. High glycemic foods such as simple carbohydrates raise blood glucose and, insulin levels and, facilitate glycogen synthesis. The remaining carbohydrates should be derived from other natural resources, such as the complex and, simple carbohydrates found in fruits, vegetables, cereals, pasta and, rice. It should be noted that when these carbohydrates are combined with other nutrients, such as protein or fat, it changes the glycemic index.

Glycemic index is a crucial aspect when it comes to weight management.

Foods with low glycemic index take time to metabolize and, deliver calories for a longer period of time. This definitely help you in your goals.

Here is the list of foods with different glycemic index

High Glycemic foods (greater than 85)

Honey, corn syrup, bagel, wheat bread, cornflakes, raisins, potato, sweet corn

Moderate Glycemic Index (60 – 85)

Spaghetti, oatmeal, banana, grapes, oranges, rice, yams, baked beans

Low glycemic foods (less than 60)

Apple, applesauce, cherries, dates, figs, peaches, pears, plums, kidney beans, chick peas, green peas, navy beans, red lentils, whole milk, skim milk, plain yogurt

Actual calculations with an example

Now you have calculated the total amount of calories you have to take

Let us take an example:

Let us consider a 30 year old, 80 kg male with height 5 feet 10 inches, let's name his as Mr. X

Now by the above mentioned formulae

For Males

(Weight in pounds x 6.23) +(height in inches x 12.7) – (age x 6.8) + 66 = Basal metabolic rate

Basal metabolic rate of X is = (176 x 6.23) + (70 x 12.7) – (30x6.8) + 66

1096 + 889 – 204 + 66 = 1847

Let's assume his activity level is sedentary – 1847 x 1.2 (activity factor) = 2216 calories

His calorie requirement is 2216 calories for stable weight management

Let's assume he want to lose some weight

Then we will put him to 500 calorie deficit a day

In that case his total calorie intake is 1716 calories.

One more formulae I have given

Here Bodyweight x 2.2 x 10 (if he want to lose weight) – 80x2.2x10 = 1760 calories

SO as you can see the total calories in both the formulae is nearly the same

Let's take it as 1725 calories as his daily intake

Now let us calculate the macros – protein, fats and, carbohydrates

1. Protein – 1 gram per bodyweight = 80 grams x 4 = 320 calories

2. Fats 20% of the total calories = 345 calories divided by 9 = 38.3 grams of fat

3. Carbohydrates – 1725 – 320 – 345 = 1060 divided by 4 = 265 grams

So,

Protein – 80 grams and, 320 calories

Fats – 38.3 grams and, 345 calories

Carbohydrates – 265 grams and, 1060 calories

This will be the total calorie distribution.

While designing the diet plan, the calorie charts can be referred and, the food list can be prepared as per the calorie distribution.

Calorie chart of commonly used Indian food

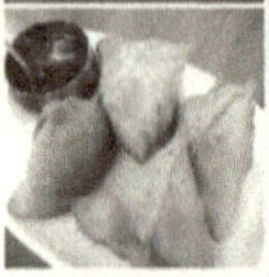

Snacks	Name	Quantity	Calories	Name	Quantity	Calories	Meat / Poultry
	Burger	1 pcs	325	Chicken	1 cup	220	
	Pizza	1 portion	375	Tandoori Chicken	2 pcs	450	
	Samosa/Kachori	1 pcs	256	Mutton (Boiled)	1 cup	100	
	Pakoda	1 pcs	200	Fish (Boiled)	1 cup	100	
	Potato Chips	10 pcs	110	Crab	1 cup	33	
	Dahi Wada	1 pcs	364	Egg (Fried)	1 pcs	100	
	French Fries	10 pcs	235	Omlette	1 pcs	110	

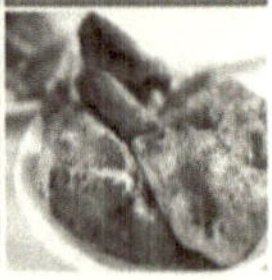

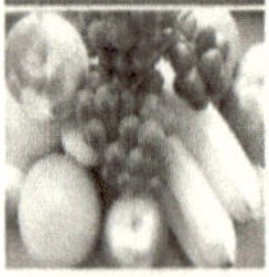

Fruits	Name	Quantity	Calories	Name	Quantity	Calories	Bread / Rice
	Apple	100 gms	56	Bread	1 slice	60	
	Banana	100 gms	95	Chapati	1 pcs	100	
	Mangoes	100 gms	70	Parantha	1 pcs	280	
	Orange	100 gms	53	Rice	100 gms	325	
	Chikoo	100 gms	94	Wheat Flour	100 gms	341	
	Papaya	100 gms	32	Maize Flour	100 gms	355	
	Peach	100 gms	50	Veg. Oil	1 tbsp	130	

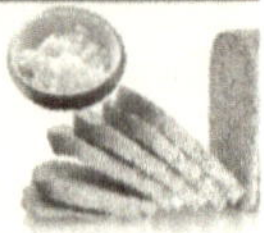

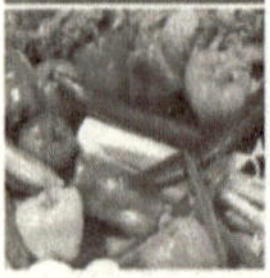

Vegetables	Name	Quantity	Calories	Name	Quantity	Calories	Sweets / Misc
	Potato	100 gms	97	Barfi	1 pcs	100	
	Peas	100 gms	93	Gulab Jamun	1 pcs	100	
	Cauliflower	100 gms	30	Jalebi	1 pcs	200	
	Cabbage	100 gms	45	Rasgulla	1 pcs	150	
	Carrot	100 gms	48	Sugar	1 tbsp	60	
	Mushroom	100 gms	18	Honey	1 tbsp	30	
	Onion	100 gms	50	Jam	1 tbsp	100	

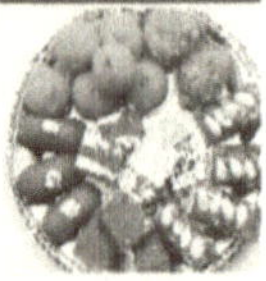

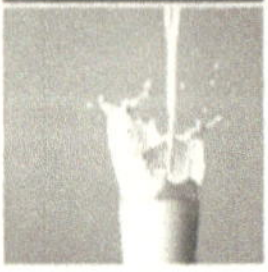

Milk & Milk Pdts	Name	Quantity	Calories	Name	Quantity	Calories	Drinks / Beverages
	Milk	1 cup	100	Cold Drinks	1 bottle	95	
	Skimmed Milk	1 cup	45	Orange Juice	1 glass	95	
	Curd	1 cup	60	Apple Juice	1 glass	95	
	Butter	1 tbsp	120	Beer	1 glass	100	
	Cheese	1 cup	164	Whisky	1 peg	75	
	Ice-Cream	1 scoop	114	Rum	1 peg	75	
	Ghee	100 gms	910	Tea/Cofee	1 cup	35	

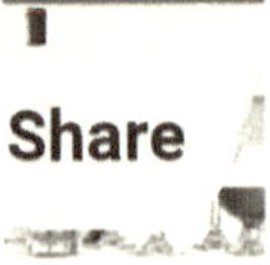

When to eat?

Timings of food and, itsimportance

Now when we have the total calories and, the calorie distribution the task is to distribute the calories in the entire day

Continuing with the above example –

Total calories are 1725 calories.

As per the traditional approach we take 3 big meals and, rest are considered to be the fillers.

Fillers can be taken between 50 to 150 calories each – we have 4 fillers – that makes it approx 500 calories on an average.

The big meals are left with 1225 calories and, each meal will consist of approx 375 calories each that is breakfast, lunch and, dinner.

There is a big debate about the quantity and, the type of food to be taken at the time of dinner.

Let me here clear it out that the total calories in the day matters, it's not a particular meal that will define your fitness goals. Please consider this point seriously.

Here I am giving you a calorie distribution for reference

Meal 1 – Immediately when you wake up or within ½ an hour of waking up (6.30am) – 100 calories

Meal 2 – Breakfast - 8.30am- 9.30 am - 350 calories

Meal 3 – Mid Morning – 11.30am to 12pm – 150 calories

Meal 4 – Lunch 1.30- 2.30 pm – 450 calories

Meal 5 - Evening – 5pm to 5.30 pm – 150 calories

Meal 6– Dinner – 8pm to 8.30 pm - 425 calories

Meal 7 – 10 pm – 100 calories

What to eat?

We all know, that we are what we eat.

As with the above calorie distribution, you have understood by now, that it's not a particular diet or food or a particular macro that can help you to reach your fitness goals but, all the macros in right proportion and, that too with variety having all the micros in them will make you not only fit but keep you healthy throughout your life time.

When it comes to fitness or health as I have seen the first meal that springs to mind is the dreaded salad, but even salad is missing important components for a healthy meal. To some eating lots and, lots of protein with some fats is considered as a complete meal and, road to achieving fitness goals, my friends without carbohydrates it's really not possible.

All the macro nutrients proteins, carbohydrates and, fats in right proportion are the energy giving components of our foods and, help our bodies to function properly. Micro nutrients on the other hand are the essential vitamins, minerals, antioxidants, and, phyto chemicals within these macro nutrients. If you reduce any of the macros you will definitely be sacrificing some of the micros also. For example if you are not taking fats, the fat soluble vitamins like vitamin K won't be absorbed easily. Experts say if you are eating unbalanced meals you will possibly gain or lose weight in an undesirable and, unhealthy way.

It is easy for me to give a diet chart but I know a particular diet chart or charts can be followed for a week, for a month or for three months maximum.

Here I give you a basic thumb rule, so that you will be able to plan your meals as per your own convenience.

In maximum of your meals try having a proportion of fats, carbohydrates and, proteins exactly same as the proportion of these macros in your total calories.

Like in the example of Mr. X –

Protein percentage in total diet = (320 / 1725) x 100 = 18.5%

Fat percentage in total diet = (345/1725) x 100 = 20%

Carbohydrate percentage in total diet = (1060/1725) x 100 = 61.5%

This is the calorie distribution of the total diet.

Now at least in the big meals this percentage should be followed

Like we have assumed breakfast to be 350 calories

Now the calorie distribution of this meal is as follows

Protein – 65 calories /4 = 16.25 grams

Fats – 70 calories /9 = 7.75 grams

Carbohydrates – 215 calories /4 = 54 grams

I suggest following for this meal

Food	Carbohydrate	Protein	Fat
2 slice bread	30grams	5.4 grams	
1 tbsp peanut butter		6 grams	8 grams
3 egg whites		10.5 grams	
150 ml fresh	20 grams		
Unsweetened juice			
TOTAL	56 grams	16 grams	8 grams

This combination solves our purpose.

Exactly, like this only we have to distribute our calories in the all the meals.

we are giving some sample diet plans for reference

Sample meal plan for 1500 calories

Meal-1

Tea/ Coffee/ Green Tea (with little or no sugar)

Meal-2

1 Bowl of sprouts of beans with low fat paneer/cheese/tofu

OR

2 Egg whites with low fat paneer/tofu/cheese

Meal-3

Vegetable sabzi + 2 roti (no butter)+ Dal rice+ Buttermilk

OR

Low fat paneer sabzi + 2 rotis (no butter) + Buttermilk

OR

1 Vegetable and, cheese whole wheat sandwich (no butter)

OR

1 Egg omelet with two whole wheat bread toasts

Meal-4

Mix fruit dish (Banana, watermelon, orange, apple etc.)

OR

1 Bowl fruit yogurt (no sugar or added flavours)

OR

1 Glass mix fruit lassi (very less sugar)

Meal-5

Baked potatoes and, vegetable chopped tomato and, onion gravy

OR

1 Glass vegetable soup with two whole wheat toasts

OR

1 Bowl brown rice with vegetable soup

Meal- 6

1 Glass low fat milk (no sugar)

Sample meal plan for 1000 Calorie Plan

Early morning

Honey, lemon juice and, warm water

OR

Apple cider vinegar and, warm water

Breakfast

Oatmeal with strawberries

Pre-Lunch

Green Tea

Lunch

Cabbage soup and, 100g low fat yogurt

Post-Lunch

1 Peach and, 1 orange

Evening Snack

Green tea and, 2 digestive biscuits

Dinner

1 Bowl of boiled lentils with stir fried French beans, capsicum and, peas with a little chopped garlic.

Nutrition before, during and, after your work out

This section I am specially writing, as we need to take care of certain things, so that we get the most benefit from a work out, whether the work out is related to strength, flexibility or endurance. In order to reap the benefits of each specific work out, it is important that you take care of appropriate nutrition and, hydration habits before, during and, after a work out session.

Pre Work out Nutrition – In order to have the most energy to complete the desired work out, it is crucial to practice appropriate and, beneficial pre-work out nutrition habits.

The pre-exercise meal is important for two reasons.

1. It prevents you from feeling hungry and, sluggish before or during a work out.

2. Second, it assists in maintaining optimal levels of energy in the form of blood glucose for exercising muscles during the work out.

Although the energy produced by food is necessary in order to perform well, it is also important to remember that exercise should not be performed on a full stomach. That is why the quantity and, quality of the food and, the time difference between pre work out meal and, work out should be utmost taken care.

Pre work out meal 1 (an hour or two before work out)

1. Whole grain cereal with non fat milk and, piece of fruit
2. Fruit shake with 100% fruit juice and, low fat yogurt
3. Ban muffin and, low fat yogurt
4. Whole grain toast with peanut butter
5. String cheese, whole grain crackers and, grapes
6. Fig newtons and, non fat chocolate milk
7. Lean turkey on whole wheat bread with an apple.

Pre work out meal 2 (30minutes before work out)

1. Whole wheat toast with jam'
2. A piece of fruit
3. Low fat yogurt
4. Non sweetened dry cereal
5. Fat free chocolate milk
6. Energy bar

During Work out – Whether you are a professional athlete who trains rigorously for a long time or you have low to moderate routine, keep your body hydrated with small, frequent sips of water.

You need not to eat during a work out that's an hour or less, but for longer, high-intensity vigorous work outs you may eat 50-100 calories every half hour of carbohydrates such as low fat yogurt, raisins, or banana.

Post Work out Nutrition – Peak performance nutrition does not only apply to pre work out food consumption, but to post work out nutrition as well. The appropriate post work out meal assist in replenishing the muscles as blood flow to muscles increases immediately after exercises, which allows the muscle cells to absorb more glucose which ultimately maximizes glycogen synthesis within the muscles. Muscles are the most receptive to recovery during the first 30 minutes after a work out. It is really important to consume protein in addition to a source of carbohydrates after exercise to repair the muscle damage that inevitably occurs following a work out. If muscle damage is not recovered or repaired after a work out, muscle glucose uptake and, muscle glycogen storage may be at risk for impairment, thus limiting your performance during the next performance and, consequently will affect reaching your goals.

Post work out Meal samples

1. Peanut butter and, banana sandwich on whole wheat bread.

2. Non-fat chocolate milk

3. Fruit shake made with banana, strawberries, mango and, 100% fruit juice and, non-fat yogurt

4. Beans and, brown rice

5. Protein shakes

6. Cereal and, non-fat yogurt

7. Turkey and, cheese on whole wheat bread

8. Pasta with lean meat spaghetti sauce

9. Peanut butter and, apple slices.

Foods to avoid around the work outs

1. Caffeine

2. Candy

3. Doughnuts and, pastries

4. Greasy food high in fat (fried chicken or fish, pizza, french fries)

5. Fructose, high fructose corn syrup

6. Highly sugared, refined cereals

7. Milk shakes and, ice creams

CHAPTER 6

EVALUATING THE PROGRESS AND, HOW TO MOVE AHEAD

Evaluating the progress and, how to move further

Rome was not built in a day.

In my entire fitness career, 99.99% people I have come across people who want to bet fit, always talk about results and, not performance or progression.

On day one, when I meet someone who want to be fit in near future, there first question is

In how much time I will be fit?

And, after nearly thirty years of consistent work out I think – am I fit enough?

Yes as we started we will only look fit if we will be fit and, there is no short cuts for it. Seriously there is not.

Why do people don't get desired results

I have really seen in person, many people who have been doing work outs for years, but there is no improvement. It's not that they do not work hard, yes, it's not so, but

1. They do not have a direction or goal – First thing to assess is, which way you have to go. What is your ultimate goal? Why have you started this program? What do you want to achieve?

a.   Do want to set your internal body parameters in place, are you going for basic health

b.   Are you looking forward to physical fitness to improve your daily activities

c.   Do you want to lose weight

d.   Do you want to overcome your injuries or joint pains

e.   Do you want to get fit for a particular sport.

f.   Do you want to take fitness as your profession.

g.   Or all of the above or any other?

Yes, the goal is really important. Then only you can make a strategy for it. Every day you have to remember that you have a particular goal and, you have to work accordingly. If you are aiming to improve your endurance there is no point doing strength training daily, or vice versa. Also your work out plan, your diet and, day to day activities should be according to your goals. It is really important to know what you want from your work out?

2.   They are not consistent - Many a times we see that when we start some activity, we are highly motivated for the work outs, diet plans and, all the respected things, but with time we are not really consistent about it. Either we do not do the work outs with the same intensity or we do not keep track with our calories. This leads to distraction and, we are not able to keep the pace with our progress and, get dishearten with time.

3.   They do not assess themselves on regular basis – Regular personal assessment is really important. Yes, when it comes to endurance a continuous check up with the time, speed and, the intensity of the work out is really important. In every work out, yes every second time when you perform that activity you have to be better than the earlier one, may be.001%, it is really important, same is the case with strength and, flexibility.

4. They do not have a clearly defined goal – This is a very important aspect, I have seen many people who do not have a concrete goal. When I ask them what do you want from the work out or this fitness regime, either the answer is I want to lose weight or I want to get fit or I want to reduce my waist line. These goals are not exact and, defined and, most specifically they do not define the plan of action.

5. They do not have patience – Last but not the least, is the patience, yes it's the most important aspect. Tell me one thing, when you took 10 or 20 odd years to gain that fat in your body then how can you even imagine of removing the fat in days or months. Body Transformation takes time, as mentioned earlier it is easy to remove water from the body and, some amount of muscle weight can be reduced by long term fasting but to remove fat takes a lot of hard work, planned diet and, yes above all patience. You have to wait for the right things to happen.

To have a clear goal is important

Every one want to get fit, I agree but the approaches and, the final goals are really different. For some fitness is getting a six pack abdominals, for some fitness is to run a marathon, fitness can also be performing well in a sport or it can just to be disease free for some.

So first thing is to have a clear goal

1. I want to get fit.

2. I want to lose 5kg weight

3. I want to lose 5kg fat weight.

4. I want to lose 5 kg fat weight in three months

5. I want to lose 5 kg fat weight in three months by doing 40 minutes jogging thrice a week and, twice a week some strength training with yoga.

6. I want to lose 5 kg fat weight in three months by doing 40 minutes jogging thrice a week and, twice a week some strength training

with yoga and, will maintain a calorie difference of 500 calories per day and, take protein fats and, carbohydrates as per my body type and, requirements.

All the above 6 statements are correct, but the sixth statement is a perfect statement. It states a goal and, the strategy to accomplish the goal. That is really important.

I am sure after reading all the previous chapters you will clearly define your goal as it is done above in statement 6.

Now when you have started with Body Transformation, lets recall the parameters you analyzed when you started the project that is "Body Transformation"

1. *Calculating the body fat percentage*
2. *Internal body parameters and, hormonal functions were analyzed.*
3. *Understanding the present Physical parameters*
   a. *Endurance*
   b. *strength*
   c. *flexibility*
4. *work out program design*
5. *Meal Planning*

You started with all the above, now its time to review, plan or re schedule certain things as per our development and, results. If we are getting better then we need to intensify or maintain the plan of action and, in case we are not then we need to assess all the parameters and, plan them accordingly.

Now, after at least a month all the above parameters need to be reevaluated and, checked. Let us discuss all of them

Analysing the body fat percentage changes

As discussed body mass is divided in two –

Fat mass and, the fat free mass (muscle mass)

Over a period of time body has taken a shape and, also gained some percentage of fat and, muscle. Now when you have started an exercise program and, also started calculating the calories also, Your weighing scale will show variation, either your weight will increase or decrease. But here I would say that the figures shown by the weighing scale are really confusing, they does not tell you what is happening inside the body.

Why do weight increase when we start an exercise program

If your goal is weight loss, and, after starting your Program, your weight increases, you will be in a great shock. Am I correct? The first thought which comes in mind is now you are exercising and, taking care of the diet also then why is your weight increasing. This condition is really demotivating. Actually people who want to lose fat, weighing scale is like the first and, the last criteria for them. If after starting a fitness program, weight increases, then it is really depressing. Let me make it really clear, it is not so. There are several research-backed reasons why you might notice a slight weight gain after exercise. Possible explanations include muscle weight gain, water retention, post-work out inflammation, supplement use, or even undigested food.

Muscle weight gain

It is likely that you will gain muscle when you start working out. How *much* muscle you gain depends on your diet and, the type of work outs you do. But any increase in physical activity is likely to produce at least some improvements in strength and, muscle mass,[1] especially if you were mostly sedentary prior to the start of your program.[2] If you are participating in strength training work outs and, you're consuming adequate protein, you're likely to see greater increases in muscle mass.

Genetics also play a role in the amount of muscle mass you gain when starting an exercise program. Some people put on muscle more easily than others. If you tend to gain muscle easily, consider yourself lucky. Muscles help to shape a strong, healthy body.

But when you gain muscle, the number on the scale is likely to increase. In fact, even if you're also losing fat, you may see an increase on the scale. Muscle is more dense than fat, but it takes up less space. That means if you gain muscle, your scale weight may go up even as you're losing body fat.

If you've been working out regularly, it's possible for you to lose inches even if you're not losing weight. A higher number on the scale could mean that you are losing fat while gaining muscle—a positive trend that leads to a leaner, stronger body.

Water weight gain

Water retention is a common cause of temporary weight gain. Pre-menopausal women are especially prone to body-weight fluctuations throughout the month due to hormonal changes.

Women are likely to notice some degree of bloating immediately before and, during their menstrual period. Exercise can help to reduce symptoms of PMS—so it's helpful to keep up with your work outs,[3] though you may still see an increase on the scale.

Studies have shown that fluid retention peaks on the first day of menstrual flow. It is lowest during the mid-follicular period (the middle phase of your cycle) and, then gradually increases over the 11 days surrounding ovulation.[4] The degree to which you see an increase on the scale varies from person to person, but at least a slight increase in weight—even after exercise—is normal.

Another common reason for water weight gain is an increase in your sodium intake. According to research, consuming high salt foods can cause an increase in bodyweight. Studies have shown that after we eat salty foods, we increase our water intake but we do not necessarily produce more urine. The extra fluid in your body adds up to pounds on the scale.[5] Some people are very sodium-sensitive and, may retain more water.

Keep in mind that even if you aren't adding salt to your food, it may still be lurking in the processed foods and, beverages that you consume.

Post-work out inflammation

It's possible that your work out itself is causing weight gain—at least temporarily. But this increase may be an indicator that you are exercising hard enough to see real results.

Very simply put, exercise (especially weight training) damages muscle tissue. The repair process that occurs after exercise allows your muscles to grow and, get stronger. But in the meantime, inflammation occurs in the tissues. Exercise physiologists call this exercise-induced muscle damage (EIMD).

EIMD is a temporary phenomenon that occurs after new or exceptionally challenging exercise patterns. It causes structural damage to myofibers (cells in muscle tissue); inflammation results due to a build-up of white blood cells in the damaged tissues.[6] This inflammation and, build-up of fluid may show up as temporary weight gain after a work out.

How do you know if your body is experiencing EIMD? You may feel DOMS, that is delayed onset of muscle soreness. You're likely to feel increased soreness the day after or even two days after your work out as a result of the inflammation and, repair that is happening in the body.

Supplement use

Post-work out nutrition or supplement use may also cause a certain degree of weight gain after working out.

Exercise—particularly prolonged endurance exercise like running or cycling—depletes the body of glycogen. It's very common for trained athletes to consume supplement beverages after exercise that contain carbohydrates. Carbs help to restore muscle glycogen. But for each gram of glycogen stored, the body retains three grams of water.[7] The result? An increase in stored water and, possible water weight gain following your work out.

Of course, this post-work out effect doesn't just apply to carbohydrate supplementation. Even carbs that you consume in meals and, snacks following your work out will be stored as glycogen with water. This is a normal and, healthy process of recovery—so it is not something you should try to avoid.

Undigested, fiber-rich food

If your work outs make you hungry and, you are refueling with healthy fiber-rich foods, the nutritious food you consume may lead to an increase in the scale as it works its way through your body.

Fiber is said to aid in water retention in the colon and, results in stools that are less dry and, easier to evacuate. Insoluble fiber, in particular, is known to increase stool weight.[11] Before the stool is passed, you might notice an increase in weight after your work out, but fiber also decreases colonic transit time, so this is not a nutrient you should avoid.

Should you worry about post-work out weight gain?

In many cases, there is no reason to worry about an increase in weight after exercise. In fact, if the weight gain is the result of one of the common causes listed above, you should take it as a sign of success.

Of course, there are other reasons that you may see an increase on the scale. Some medications may cause weight gain or your calorie intake may have increased along with your hunger levels after exercise. You need to keep a check on it.

It may be helpful to use methods other than the scale to measure your work out progress to figure out if changes if warranted.

So as you can see you need not worry, if there is a sudden increase in the bodyweight, when you started your exercise program. You need to analyse the changes as given below.

Now let us see how to analyze the changes in weighing scale –

Case 1 – Weight is constant

In this case three possibilities are there

    a. There is no change in the muscle mass or the fat mass that means there is no difference between the calories you are burning and, taking. You need to put in more efforts and, create a calorie difference. Here it is a good sign that the weight is not increasing that means the body is in a positive state.

b. Your muscle weight is increasing and, the fat weight is decreasing, this is a real positive sign and, that is what is required. Good work.

c. Your fat weight is increasing and, your muscle weight is decreasing, this is really bad and, you need to check the diet and, work out goingon.

Case 2 – Weight is increasing

Here there are two possibilities

a. Muscle weight is increasing, all the possibilities have been just discussed above.

b. Fat weight is increasing – Yes, this can be a possibility, when we are not burning enough calories and, also at the same time taking calories more than we are burning. In that case body is storing calories as fat. Also there can be many internal body parameters also which need time to get into place, so keep observing the pattern and, take proper corrective measures and, also try maintaining the calorie deficit.

Case 3 – When weight is decreasing

a. Fat weight is decreasing – In this case it is clear that you are successful in maintaining the calorie deficit and, the fitness program is going good. Just carry on and, do maintain your protein count so that the muscle weight does not decrease.

b. Muscle Weight is decreasing – This is the most dangerous situation, it indicates that you are over training and, at the same time the calorie count has been drastically reduced and, you are fasting, in this case body does not loses fat, it just lose muscle mass and, water. Take immediate action.

I agree Bodyweight is important, but when it comes to body transformation, body composition is utmost important. In the starting period you should be more conscious about the body composition. Your goal should be reducing the fat percentage and, maintaining or increasing the muscle mass unless and, until, your primary goal is to reduce weight. If your goal is to reduce bodyweight any how, in that case also I would not recommend losing the muscle mass drastically as this is not good and, will take your body in negative and, SOS mode and, that lost weight will definitely be temporary and, it will come back.

Now as we started, we checked our body fat percentage by following methods:

1. Body Composition analysis
2. Calculating the body mass index
3. Waist hip ratio
4. Skin fold test
5. Under water weighing

Now as your bodyweight varies, after a period of time, like a month or so, you should again get your body composition checked by any of the above means and, keep a record of it. This analysis will tell you, that what is the actual reason of the bodyweight variations. Is it the muscle mass or the fat mass. When you get to know the reason, you will be able to easily change, maintain, or intensify your diet and, training plan. It is the exact way.

Analysing the internal body parameters changes by blood tests

Now the second aspect we checked was the internal body parameters and, the hormonal functions –

Here I will mention, that when it comes to fitness and, body transformation, we always talk about only work out and, diet, but the internal body parameters play a major role and, they can definitely govern the entire situation. Yes I agree that with time when you will work out and, take care of your diet certain your metabolism and, certain body functions will definitely improve but there are certain complications which can create trouble and, inspite of all the efforts, results will not be what you are looking for or they will take unexpected time.

When we started the program, we got our blood tests done and, all the reports were to be analyzed properly and, the corrective measures were taken. (all the corrective measures are mentioned in chapter 8)

Now after a month or 45 days we have to get our blood tests again done, either all the tests or atleast the test which were not up to the mark.

By this action we will get to know that what are the changes happening inside the body, by our fitness program.

Let us discuss them one by one –

1. Lipid Profile test which told us about the cholesterol levels inside the body.

   If you had Higher bad cholesterol levels (LDL) and, higher Triglyceride levels, then you must have stopped taking the bad fats and, also increased the endurance activities as mentioned.

   Now when you will again get this test done you will come to know how much improvement is there and, if the problem is still the same or marginally better then you have to take intense actions like further monitoring your diet and, do the cardio vascular activities in intense manner taking care of the target heart rate.

   Also you need to check the HDL, that is good cholesterol, is it up to the mark and, if not then, you need to take good fats in an adequate manner as it is a really important factor, where it helps in fat burning and, increasing the immunity, it also help in controlling the reproductive hormones which can affect your muscle mass and, hence metabolism.

2. Gastro Intestinal Tract – Here we checked the ESR (erythrocyte sedimentation rate), C-Reactive Protein, Homo cysteine.

   It is important to check, how is the intestine and, related body parts working. These parameters clearly indicates, if there is any inflammation inside the body or there is some kind of leakage, due to which food digestion will not be proper and, also the nutrients will not be stored. Getting this test again will clear the picture and, you can take the necessary action.

3. Thyroid Gland - The most important gland, when it comes to body transformation and, weight management. It directly affects our goals as the hormones secreted by this gland controls the body metabolism and, digestive functions.

   We need to check all the Thyroid functioning parameters, T3, T4, TSH and, others, which will help you to keep track and, take required nutrients or medications if required.

4. Insulin Resistance – As discussed earlier, Insulin controls the amount of sugar or glucose in blood and, insulin resistance is a disease when the body's cells does not accept the glucose.

   This was checked by testing Fasting Insulin, Fasting blood glucose, HBA1C. Now this is a real critical factor, it need to be checked timely as it can really alter your blood glucose levels and, you may face a problem called insulin spike. Also if this problem persist than the foods with high glycemic index will not help, which are generally considered to be light and, helping in weight management. You have to keep a strict eye on all three, and, get it checked with time.

5. Liver, Here we examined the SGPT and, SGOT levels which clearly shows the liver toxicity, now we need to get it regularly checked till these parameters come below 20. It is really important to be monitored.

6. Kidney functioning test- Uric acid and, other kidney parameters need to be monitored as they play an important role in body transformation.

7. Adrenaline gland functioning and, the cortisol levels need to be continuously monitored as it disturbs our metabolism, immune system, blood pressure and, response to stress.

In all the above aspects, it is really difficult to continue with our body transformation goals. We need to get our cortisol levels checked and, take the nutrients and, diet accordingly.

8. Our reproductive hormones, now we need to check that after starting our fitness program what is the effect on them. Now re they in acceptable ranges and, if not, it need to be taken care as they controls the muscle development and, fat reduction.

9. Vitamins and, Minerals, the micro nutrients, were checked when we started the program. This point is really critical. In maximum of the cases I have seen when people start the fitness program, they get really strict about their diet. In this case there is definitely a possibility, if diet is not planned taking care of all the nutrients then, several nutrients will be in deficit, which will be really harmful for our metabolism and, hormones, Here I ll mention that if this happens we will be in a negative state and, we will never be able to achieve our goals. So I strongly recommend to get the micro nutrients regularly checked.

10. Food Allergies and, Toxicity: You need to get it checked again, regarding the food allergies, as it will definitely help in meal planning and, also reduce the possibility of stomach inflammation and, discomfort helping in proper digestion and, fat loss.

I would mention here that if you are really serious about your body transformation the internal parameters can never be ignored. They really need to be taken care, by all means

a. They need to be checked after regular intervals of time.

b. Proper diet alterations and, work out manipulations should be done accordingly

c. All the macros, micros and, super foods as per the reports need to taken

d. If necessary proper nutrients, medications or supplementation should also be taken.

Analysing the physical parameters and, importance of progression

I agree it takes a lot to start a fitness regime, and, also all the above discussion shows, it is equally important to evaluate the results and, the progress.

The word "Progression" is really important in Body Transformation.

I may put it as "Better than before" or continuous improvement.

Let's take an example

Case 1

Mr. Ram want to improve his strength, he started a fitness program. After a week or fifteen days he was able to do 10 pushups, 5 pull ups, 20 squats. Then after a month he did 10 pushups, 4 pull ups and, 20 squats. Then he continued with the program and, diet regime and, after 2 months he did 8 push-ups, 4 pull ups and, 18 squats.

Case 2

Mr. Ram want to improve his strength, he started a fitness program. After fifteen days he was able to do 15 pushups, 6 pull ups, 20 squats. Then after a month he did 18 pushups, 8pull ups and, 30 squats. Then he continued with the program and, diet regime and, after 2 months he did 20 push-ups, 11 pull ups and, 36 squats.

In Case 1 as you can see the performance is either the same or it's decreasing but in Case 2 performance is getting better with time. This shows that in Case 2 Mr. Ram is progressive, he is doing his work outs seriously, putting all the efforts in his training and, at the same time he is taking care of his balanced diet with good amount of protein, carbohydrates and, fats.

So, if you really want your body transformation program to work, you need to assess your progress each single day.

Let us take another example

Miss Sushma is going for jogging thrice a week. In first week she did 3.5km in 45 minutes, in second week she was able to cover 4km in 45 minutes and, after a month she did 5km in 45 minutes.

This shows progression.

Yes, this is the way it works. We have to put efforts in every work out. Like while doing strength work outs, if we did 12 repetitions with a 10 kg dumbbell than we should definitely keep a record of all the weights and, the repetitions in all the exercises, and, every time we do the exercise, it should be better than the earlier work out in terms of weights or repetitions.

What is exercise plateau and, how to tackle it

When we are talking about the physical parameters it is really important to discuss about the word

Exercise plateau or the saturation level.

Many a times it happens you will feel like you have hit a road block in your fitness journey, I agree this happens to most of the people.

A work out plateau occurs when your body adjusts to the demands of your work outs. To keep seeing results, you need to progressively overload the body to keep it changing, adapting and, getting stronger. Just because your work outs are getting easier does not mean you have hit a plateau although it can feel that way. When you start any new form of training, it can take around six to eight weeks for the brain and, body to learn to complete new exercise efficiently. Once these changes are adapted, the work outs should feel easier. This is not work out plateau, as you continue to build muscular strength and, endurance.

During a work out plateau, you may start to feel unmotivated, bored with your work outs which indirectly will affect your results and, the goals and, you may also feel that you are not getting better or progressing.

Why this happens?

a. When you first start working out you usually feel results or good changes in your body, especially if you were not active previously.

However as time passes and, your body adjust to exercising you may notice the results less obvious.

The body adapts to the physical demands of the training. As your body adapts, exercises that were once challenging, becomes easier. This is why you can hit a plateau even when you are doing everything right.

b. Another common cause of a plateau is over training. Getting proper rest and, recovery is just as important for your fitness progress as hitting all of your work outs. Signs that you are overtraining include muscle and, joint pain, fatigue or low energy levels. You may find that you get sick more easily.

c. Also you can stop making progress if you do not take care of your diet and, water intake.

Now what is important is your fitness goals, if you are happy with your current fitness levels, keep going with your current exercise routine to maintain fitness. However if you are frustrated with the lack of progress do not despair.

There are actions you can take to overcome this fitness plateau

a. Making changes to your work outs can help prevent a plateau and, increase results also. In case of strength training, when you increase the weight, sets, reps, intensity, number of sessions completed each week, the amount of rest taken sets or sue variations of your exercises you encourage a training response to occur. Making small changes regularly encourages your body to building strength using the same exercise. Some examples of fitness progression include

1. Increasing reps of an exercise with same weight or increasing bit weight and, doing same reps

2. Increasing the speed in an endurance training or reducing the time and, covering same distance

3. In case of circuit training or HIIT training completing the exercise schedule in lesser time or increasing the number of exercises completed in a given time frame.

    4. You may increase the level of your training, from beginner to intermediate or from intermediate to advance, challenge yourself in a progressive mode.

b. Track your fitness progress – You can not be sure you have hit a plateau unless you are tracking your progress. Like

    1. Record your work outs, including the number of reps and, weights

    2. You may use a fitness tracker – record your RHR, THR,

    3. Take progress photos

    4. Take a timed fitness challenges every 4 weeks, like if you are into endurance training, you may do 5k or 10k run once in a month to challenge yourself. In strength training you can do 1 Rep maximum in certain exercises to check your strength and, keep check on it

Tracking your fitness can help you identify whether you are in a plateau and, what you can change to overcome it.

c. Resistance training or strength training, improves strength, endurance and, size of skeletal muscles while protecting your joints from injury during other activities. Muscles burns more energy than fat, so building lean muscle can help boost your metabolic rate. Resistance training also helps with cardiovascular health, particularly if you combine it with cardio. Strength training can help you to achieve other goals such as running faster, or improving your sport, or skin tone up and, spot reduction.

d. Focus on Nutrition – Nutrition plays an important role in your fitness progress and, to keep improving, you need a nutrition plan that supports your training. This means getting enough macros and, micros are really important to build muscle and, recover quickly. Also good hydration plays a critical role in muscle performance and, recovery. It also plays an essential role in your heart health and, your digestive system.

e. Make time for rest – Rest days allow you to take a break from training and, allow your body to recover. During rest, your body begins to replenish its energy stores and, when it gets to work repairing the muscle tissue used during the work outs. This is an essential part of the process to progress further towards your goals.

f. Be serious with your flexibility routines – You need to practice your stretching and, flexibility routines regularly and, as scheduled. It helps in relaxing your muscles and, joints, it lengthens the muscle fibers and, also removes all the lactic acid. It relieves you from all the body pains and, definitely increase your strength and, stamina to progress towards your goals.

Assessing the work out program design

When you started your body transformation, the initial work out program you have made was on the basis of your starting body type, the body fat percentage, all the internal body parameters.

With time, as discussed above you have to evaluate all these parameters at regular intervals and, make modifications in your work out program design to reach your goals.

Let us take an example:

Ruchi, weight 68 kg was an Endomorph, with body fat 42%.

In order to lose body fat she focused more on cardio training and, also some strength based activities and, that too in cardio or circuit form to keep her heart rate elevated. After some time with serious training and, balanced diet she lost good amount of fat. Now what she needs is to tone up also build strength. In this case as you can see the initial work out design had more of endurance training and, balanced diet, but now she will have to focus equally on endurance training as well as strength and, flexibility. Also in her diet she will have to concentrate on protein also.

Let us take another example

Aman, an ecto morph who wanted to develop strength and, gain some muscle weight, started with basic strength training, now with time he has gained good muscle mass, and, now he is looking for some total body development and, definition also. Also he want to work on some weak points also. In this case he has to definitely modify his work out program accordingly.

As I always say:

"The strategy by which you have reached this level, will not take you to the next level."

Yes it is true. With time and, present position you have to make necessary modifications in your work out program as per the goals so that you can move further.

Here I would mention that, many a times I have seen that people are not able to carry on with their work out programs. There may be many reasons like their body is not yet prepared for it, the time or place or the activity is not suiting them, they are not able to gel with the people or they are having some kind of family or peer pressure. It happens, in that case, do not get dishearten or take things negatively, never think that you cannot do it. You can always alter the program and, carry on with what you can.

Remember, in the starting it is really important to carry on with what you can rather than what you should.

In the start people ask "why you are doing it?" and, then they will ask "how you did it?"

Assessing the meal plan

Success of your body transformation program really depends on how honest you are with your diet regime.

When you started with the program you must be really adhering to the total calories, the proteins, carbohydrates, the good fats, the vitamins and, minerals, but as time passes it is, yes it is very difficult to stick to your diet plans.

There are many reasons to it but solutions are there too –

a. Availability and, affordability – Whenever it comes to diet food or the healthy food, the recipes or the foods prescribed or suggested are generally out of reach. Foods like avocados, berries, broccoli, multi colored peppers, many kind of so called super foods, condiments, imported cheese and, many others. These items are not readily available and, also for a common man they are not economically viable on daily basis. In those cases many people are not able to stick to their diet regimes.

Solution – Let me tell you it's actually not so. If you can easily get these foods then it is fine, if not, then it is not really important to do so. What matters is the amount of calories you intake, and, the calorie distribution in terms of macros. I have always advised people to stick to their staple food when it comes to body transformation.

Rule 1 – You just need to count the calories.

Rule 2 – You have to make sure you are taking in calculated amount of proteins, fats, carbohydrates.

Rule 3 – You have to follow the timing of your meals

Rule 4 – You have to avoid the high calorie foods

Rule 5 – You have to avoid all kind of bad fat foods

Rule 6 – You need to check your bodyweight and, fat % regularly

Yes trust me, it is possible with your daily staple diet, you just need to open your eyes, follow the calculations before you eat.

b. Environmental Pressure – People around, it may be our family, friends, peer group, our juniors or seniors, neighborhood, even the person whom you meet once in a month, will strongly try and, influence you, the very first day you decide to start your diet or meal planning. I really agree to this, and, really wonder why people do not encourage the one who want to follow healthy diet regime?

Every one around you will disturb you, you will have to listen to lines like:

Why are you doing this?

You don't need to do this

What is the need?

You already look good

You will get weak

Just taste this a bit

This much is fine, it won't harm

And, so on

These lines and, the surroundings creates an undue pressure and, at times we are not able to stick to our meal plans.

Solution - Yes I agree these lines are disturbing and, irritating too.

As I always say, its really easy to work out for an hour, but what you do the rest of the twenty three hours in a day, decides your success. Here it actually shows that how determined you are and, how much you are serious for your body transformation.

We have to train our mind, so that we can stick to our diet plans and, the external factors becomes negligible.

Rule1 – Just avoid such people who disturbs.

Rule 2 – Learn how to give smart answers

Rule 3 – Never try to prove yourself on such people, trust me you will never be able to convince those, who don't want to

Rule 4 – In extreme cases, if you have to eat some thing unhealthy, do not get frustrated, learn how to burn those extra calories. A cheat meal will not destroy the entire plan.

Rule 5 – keep smiling and, be gentle to people, When you will give results, they will understand and, appreciate.

c. Personal Factors – With time we develop certain tastes for fast food, sweets, high calorie snacks and, many other personal favorite munching habits, these foods will disturb us in our body transformation program. Yes they will. some are emotional eaters also. Their eating habits depends on their moods, in different moods they eat or some drink also. These habits also disturb a lot.

Solution - I agree you will not be able to stop your liking towards these foods, but slowly and, gradually you can.

Trust me, having calories is easy and, satisfying but burning calories is really painfull. You cannot burn sa many calories as many you can intake that too within no time. For example 1 cup or 100 grams French fries is approx 300 calories and, to burn 300 calories

You have to run for 40 minutes at a moderate pace.

You have to reduce the intake of the high calorie foods gradually and, keep doing your work out sincerely. The faster you will control your calories, the faster will be the results.

Will power is the key in this case, you have to be focused on your goals and, stick to your meal plan by all means.

Rule 1 – Try fixing your cheat window on weekly basis, and, gradually decrease that window to zero and, one fine day you will be in full control of your situation.

Rule 2 – Try diverting your mind when you know that you are about to cheat – read books, listen music, get busy with work or meditate etc

Rule 3 – Increase your will power, that will help

Rule 4 – make friends, who are like minded, who motivate you for your goals

Rule 5 – fix your cheat days, it can be once a week or it can also be once a day with calculated amount of calories.

When taken care of all the above mentioned aspects, gradually you will be able to stick to your meal plans.

In your meal plans also, you have to track your progress, do take care of following:

1. You have to monitor your bodyweight on regular intervals to check the calorie deficit. If your bodyweight numbers are ticking as per plans no need to exaggerate or intensify your diet. Let it go

2. Always remember you are what you eat – Eating right proportion of protein, fats and, carbohydrates will make gradual changes in your body type. With time check your body fat and, muscle percentage, so that you get to know the internal changes.

3. At times it happens that you will not feel hungry, but you have to eat as per the meal plan, or you will be in further deficit of calories, which will affect your performance in training.

4. Always take care of your pre, during and, post work out meals, they are really important.

5. When body fat % goes down you will feel bit dizzy and, weak, do not worry, it is part of the program. Just make sure you are having enough calories.

6. Take care of your water intake, it is really important.

7. When your bodyweight changes, do remember to make necessary modifications in your meal plan.

   Here I will mention, that there are certain metabolic and, hormonal factors, which need to be taken care in special cases. These we will discuss in chapter 7.

   I would insist regular monitoring is really important. I once remember going on a highway, I took a wrong road and, went 20 km, then I realized and, I have to travel back.

   It wasted lot of time and, efforts.

   Same is the case with body transformation, you have to be conscious and, alert about the proceedings then only you will achieve your targets and, that too in stipulated time period.

CHAPTER 7

HOW TO TACKLE WITH INTERNAL BODY DISORDERS

Special population with internal disorders and, the corrective measures

"Obesity, never comes alone", always remember this line.

As I said "Overweight or Obesity never comes alone", it increase the risk of many other health problems also.

Let's discuss

Gaining few kilos during the year may not seem like a big deal. But these kilos generally adds up over time. This extra weight creates lot many problems inside the body like

1. Type 2 Diabetes – Around 90% of adults with diabetes are overweight. It is not clear why people who are overweight are more likely to develop this disease. It may be that being overweight cause cells to change, making them resistant to the hormone insulin. Insulin carries sugar from blood to the cells, where it is used for energy. When a person is insulin resistant, blood sugar cannot be taken up by the cells, resulting in high blood sugar. In addition, the cells that produce insulin must work extra hard to keep blood sugar normal. This may cause these cells to gradually fail.

2. High blood pressure – A blood pressure is 120/80 mm hg is considered normal. If the top number (systolic blood pressure) is

consistently 140 or higher or the bottom number (diastolic blood pressure) is 90 or higher, you are considered to have high blood pressure. High blood pressure is linked to obesity in several ways. Having a large body size may increase blood pressure because your heart need to pump harder to supply blood to all your cells.

3. Kidney issues – Obesity increase the risk of diabetes and, high blood pressure, the most common cause of chronic kidney disease. Excess fat may also damage kidneys, which help regulate blood pressure. It is suggested by studies that obesity itself may promote kidney disease and, quicken its progress.

4. Heart Diseases - People who are overweight often have health problems that may increase the risk for heart disease. These problems include high blood pressure, high cholesterol, high blood sugar. In addition, excess weight may cause changes to your heart that make it work harder to send blood to all cells in your body. Also these symptoms or problems ae the leading cause of heart strokes.

5. Cancer – Being overweight also increases the risk of developing certain cancers, like breast (after menopause), colon and, rectum, gall bladder, kidney. Fat cells may release hormones that affect cell growth, leading to cancer.

6. Sleep Apnea – is a condition in which a person has one or more pauses in breathing during sleep. A person who is overweight may have more fat stored around the neck. This may make the air way smaller which makes breathing difficult or loud because of snoring. Also fat stored in the neck and, throughout the body may produce substances that cause inflammation.

7. Osteoarthritis - Being overweight is one of the risk factors for osteoarthritis, along with joint injury, older age and, genetic factors. Extra weight places extra pressure on joints and, cartilage, causing them to wear away. In addition, people with more body fat may have higher blood levels of substances that cause inflammation. Inflamed joints raise the risk for osteoarthritis.

8. Non-alcoholic Fatty liver disease – occurs when fat builds up in the liver and, causes injury. It lead to severe liver damage. It produces mild or no symptoms. The disease most often affects people who are middle aged, overweight or obese and, diabetic.

9. Pregnancy problems – Pregnant women who are overweight are more likely to develop insulin resistance, high blood sugar and, high blood pressure. Severe obesity increases surgery time and, blood loss also. Gaining too much weight during pregnancy can have long term effects for both mother and, child. These effects include that the mother will have obesity after the child is born, also the baby may gain too much weight in later stage.

10. Digestive issues – Obesity has been associated with a higher risk of GERD (gstroesophageal reflux disease, which occurs when stomach acid leas into the esophagus. In addition obesity increase the risk of developing gallstones. This is when the bile builds up and, hardens in the gall bladder. It also leads to intestinal permeability in which there developes a leakage in the gastro intestinal track which results in the unwanted leakages of nutrients.

11. Increase Depression – Obesity can affect your mental health, including higher risk of depression and, stress levels.

"Obesity never comes alone"

Let us come to this line once again

As you just saw that when weight increases, body has to work in an un conventional manner externally and, internally. Here, seriously speaking you look forward to curing all the health problems, doing all home remedies, take the so called "superfoods" available in the market, staring from ayurveda to homeopathy and, then finally they start with the allopathic medicines and, accept that you are ill. Yes you and, your surroundings one day will convince you that you are ill and, you need a doctor.

That day you start thinking that What happened to me, I was fine"

Sooner or later, by the time you decide for body transformation, till then you don't know, to what extent obesity has harm your external and, internal system.

Here only work out and, diet will not work, side by side you have to consider all the health problems also. Without considering these parameters, no matter how much work hard but you will not get the results as per your time frame which leads to frustration and, there is a possibility that you will give up.

Here with your work out and, diet you have to take care of the health problems which are created because of obesity.

First step is, that you have to identify all the possible problems, and, then you have to add all the corrective measures in respect to the problems you have.

Here with we are giving the possible corrective measures for all the health problems related to obesity:

1. Corrective measures for people with heart problems

Tests – Lipid Profile including HDL, LDL, Triglycerides, LDL/HDL ratio, VLDL, Total Cholestrol

All these test need to be done.

Now if your triglycerides, LDL, VLDL, Total Cholestrol are high, that means your heart health is not good. Bad cholesterol levels are high in your blood.

Effect on work out – In this case, endurance training will be a problem for you and, you will get tired early and, easily as the heart will not be able to pump enough blood in the activity area.

Work out considerations –

1. I agree that endurance training will be difficult for you, but on the contrary endurance training is the only solution for this problem. You have to do 40 to 60 minutes of cardio training at least 5 days a weak. To start with do at 40% to 50% of intensity, that means if

your age is 25, then 220 minus 26 = 194 and, 50% intensity will be 97. So you can maintain 97 heart rate. Gradually with time and, training you should go upto 80% intensity (155 heart rate)

2. Daily when you wake up from bed you will check your resting pulse. Gradually when you will train your resting heart rate will come down, that is the first sign that your bad cholesterol levels are coming down.

3. On weekly basis calculate your VO2 max, that is the capacity of your body to consume oxygen while work out. It's real important. With your traing vo2 max will increase with time showing that your heart health is increasing.

4. Remember, that the strength training and, flexibility routine you do should also be in a non stop manner so that your target heart rate is reached. You lose maximum fat at your target heart rate, never forget that.

Diet Considerations

1. First and, foremost thing, you have to stay away from saturated fats and, trans fats. Just make them zero in your daily diet. Like no read meat or any kind of processed meats, no full fat dairies, no fried foods and, also limiting cooking with oils.

2. No sugar foods and, beverages

3. Emphasizing fruits, vegetables, whole grains, poultry, fish and, nuts. (diet high in fibre).

4. No fast food

5. No smoking

Here one thing to be considered if your HDL, good cholesterol is low, its not good

In that case you have to intake foods that are high in good cholesterol like eggs, cheese, shellfish, organ meats full fat yogurt and, nuts.

Some foods that really help in lowering bad cholesterol:

Oats, barley and, other whole grains, beans, eggplant and, okra, vegetable oils like sunflower or canola or safflower, pectin rich foods like apple, grapes, strawberries, citrus fruits, foods fortified with sterols and, stenols, soy foods like tofu and, soy milk, fatty fish,

Some food supplements are also available in market to lower cholesterol

1. Fiber supplements – Psyllium husk, to be added with your meals
2. Sterols and, stenols rich foods
3. Red yeast rice
4. Artichoke leaf extract
5. Fenugreek seeds
6. Fish oil
7. Garlic
8. Ginseng
9. Guggul
10. Niacin
11. Soy protein

Combination of three of the above will help in lowering cholesterol with time, obviously when combined with work out and, balanced diet.

I strongly recommend to get your cholesterol levels checked regularly and, make the necessary changes. If the above recommendations in the work out and, diet are followed sincerely, the bad cholesterol levels will normalize with time.

2. Gastro Intestinal Tract / Inflammatory condition

Tests - ESR (erythrocyte sedimentation rate), C-Reactive Protein

Now if your values ESR values are on higher side, that means erythrocytes (red blood cells) are being settled at faster than normal rate which indicates inflammation in the body. Inflammation is part of your immune response system and, it may be a sign of a chronic disease, an immune disorder or other medical condition like arthritis or inflammatory bowel disease.

ESR can be checked when you have symptoms like headaches, fever, joint stiffness, neck or shoulder pain loss of appetite.

C-reactive protein is a substance produced by the liver in response to inflammation, high CRP levels indicate that there is inflammation inside the body and, this test results when studied with cholesterol levels can also show the heart health. High CRP levels also play a role in type 2 diabetes also. CRP levels can be used to diagnose inflammatory autoimmune disease like Inflammatory bowel disease and, rheumatoid arthritis.

The higher ESR and, CRP levels indicates that there is inflammation inside the body.

When it comes to body transformation this inflammation need to be taken care otherwise our work out will be disturbed due to joint pain and, stiffness and, also our diet have to be compromised or restricted because of the inflammation inside the body. Target this inflammation with diet and, exercise and, you should also see if there are other medical reasons for the inflammation by consulting your doctor. You will have to get these tests done at regular intervals.

I agree that with joint pain and, stiffness it is really difficult to pursue rigorous activities and, at times people with these issues are not even able to do low to moderate activities. Here I would say that physically active individuals are healthier, happier and, live longer than those who are inactive and, unfit. This is especially true for people with joint issues. Yet, joint issues is one of the most common reasons people give for limiting physical activity. Although seriously speaking inactivity, in addition to joint related problems, will result in a variety of health risks including type 2 diabetes, cardio vascular disease and, osteoporosis.

In simple words, If you will not work out the matter will get worse and, will invite many more health issues.

Work out considerations – In this case there are three levels of exercises

Level 1- Therapeutic exercises, prescribed by health professionals, address specific joints or body parts affected by the joint pains. A therapeutic exercise program is often a necessary first step for individuals who have been inactive, have restricted joint motion or muscle strength.

Level 2 - If you have never really exercised before or have a condition that keeps you away from doing rigorous activity go for a lighter work out that last for atleast 30 minutes. Even Moving a little bit each day will bring down the inflammation.

a. Like you can go for a walk at a brisk pace

b. Stretching daily can help reduce stiffness and, increase range of motion.

c. Flowing movements like yoga, gentle poses or meditation can help

d. Water exercises – water helps support bodyweight, that means that water exercises do not impact heavily on the joints. Water treadmills are also available now a days.

e. Cycling – stationary or outdoors can be a safe way to get the joints moving and, improve cardiovascular fitness

f. Strength training with a resistance band and, light weights will help to strengthen muscles around the joints, it will support the joints.

Level 3 – Starting a regular exercise program can be very challenging. You should be very cautious about the selection of the exercises that are safe and, customized to your specific needs and, also you have to monitor your body's response to exercise, and, modify your exercise routine as needed. Also you can make an exercise program in which you can primarily use the joints which are not paining or are less stiff and, give rest to the joints which are not that supportive.

Some guidelines are as follows:

a. Set realistic and, short and, long term goals, and, reward yourself when you achieve them.

b. Exercise with a partner or a professional

c. Keep an exercise diary and, track your progress

d. Identify problems or obstacles that are likely to trouble and, plan ahead to deal them

e. Choose activities that are convenient, relatively inexpensive and, fun.

Diet considerations

An anti-inflammatory diet should combine a variety of foods that are rich in nutrients, provide a range of antioxidants and, contain healthful fats.

Foods that can help manage inflammation include:

a. Oily fish like tuna and, salmon

b. Fruits, such as berries and, cherries

c. Vegetables, including kale, spinach and, broccoli

d. Beans

e. Nuts and, seeds

f. Olives and, olive oil

g. Fiber

h. Legumes, such a lentils

i. Spices such as ginger and, turmeric

j. Probiotics and, prebiotics

k. Tea and, some herbs

Please remember that no single food will help, food should be fresh not processed and, a colorful plate will provide a range of anti oxidants.

People who are following an anti-inflammatory diet should avoid the intake of:

a. Processed foods

b. Foods with added sugar or salt

c. Unhealthful oils

d. Processed carbs like white bread, white pasta and, many baked foods.

e. Processed snack foods such as chips and, crackers

f. Premade desserts such as cookies, candy and, ice cream

g. Excess alcohol

h. Limit the intake of gluten

In this case I would strongly recommend to get the food toxicity test done and, stop eating foods you are allergic too. That will definitely help.

There are may supplements available in the market that have been shown to reduce inflammation in studies

a. Alpha lipoic acid

b. Fish oil

c. Ginger and, curcumin

d. Resveratrol

e. Spirulina

f. Boswellia

g. Chondroitin

h. Flax

i. Methylsulfonylmethane

j. Quercetin

k. Turmeric

3. Thyroid Gland Malfunctioning

Test Done – T3, T4, TSH, Thyroid Antibodies, Reverse T3

The thyroid produces two major hormones triiodothyronine T3 and, thyroxine T4.

If these are not produced enough, you may experience symptoms such a s weight gain, lack of energy and, depression. This is called hypothyroidism.

If these are produced in excess, then symptoms are weight loss, high levels of anxiety, tremors. This is called hyperthyroidism.

The TSH test measures level of thyroid stimulating hormone in your blood. If you have a TSH reading above 2.0 mlU/L, you are at risk for progressing to hypothyroidism.

It has been appreciated for a very long time that there is a complex relationship between thyroid disease, bodyweight and, metabolism. If you have a thyroid disorder your bodyweight will definitely not be stable and, it will play a major role in our body transformation journey.

Work out considerations

In case of Thyroid malfunction it is not easy to work out at times. The condition can cause symptoms like weight gain or lose, fatigue, achy joints. You may experience times when you feel that you don't have the energy to move. Yet because it can help manage all symptoms, regular work out plays a vital role in your body transformation program.

Apart from weight management, regular exercise can help you to decrease joint pain, relieve depression, boost energy and, also increase muscle mass.

Link between thyroid disease and, fragile bones

Thyroid hormone affects the rate of bone replacement. Too much thyroid hormone in your body speed the rate at which bone is lost. If this happens too fast the body may not be able to replace the bone loss quickly enough. If the thyroxine levels stays too high for long period or the TSH stay low there is high risk of developing osteoporosis. This is the case of hyperthyroid.

In case of hypothyroid where the hormones are less secreted, in that case the patient take medicine to increase the thyroxine. Prolonged use of these medicines, if not monitored regularly may increase the hormone in the body abnormally and, lead to bone loss. In that case the bones become fragile and, joints achy. That need to be taken care while work out.

If you face problem with joints, you may refer the work out considerations in the inflammation section.

Link between thyroid disease and, heart health

Too little or too much of this hormone can contribute to health problems. Thyroid hormone influences the force and, speed of your heart beat, your blood pressure and, cholesterol level.

Hypothyroidism can affect the heart and, circulatory system in number of ways. Insufficient thyroid hormone slows your heart rate. Because it also makes the arteries less elastic, blood pressure rises in order to circulate blood around the body. Elevated cholesterol levels, which contribute to narrowed, hardened artries are also the consequence of low thyroid levels.

Hyperthyroidism, the opposite problem, can also harm the heart. Excess thyroid hormone causes heart to beat faster and, harder and, may trigger abnormal heart rythms. People may have high blood pressure.

Also as we saw above, how thyroid can affect heart health, endurance training should be seriously handled. As in the start it may be a trouble, in that case you may start with low to moderate intensity for 10 to 20 minutes and, then gradually increase it.

Do see your doctor for severity of the thyroid disease and, take medications if necessary, it is really important for your body transformation program.

Diet considerations

Foods alone won't thyroid disease, however, a combination of the right nutrients and, medication can help restore thyroid function and, minimize your symptoms.

Foods to avoid

a. Millet – all varieties

b. Highly processed foods – hot dogs, cakes, cookies etc

   Certain foods containing goitrogens or are known as irritants if consumed in large amounts

c. Soy based foods like tofu, beans, soy milk, tempeh

d. Cruciferous vegetables like broccoli, kale, spinach, cabbage etc

e. Certain fruits like peaches, pears and, strawberries

f. Beverages like coffee, green tea and, alcohol

Foods to eat

a.   Eggs – whole eggs are best

b.   Meats – all meats

c.   Fish – all sea food

d.   All vegetables in cooked form

e.   Fruits – all other fruits, including berries, banana, orange, tomatoes etc

f.   Gluten free grains and, seeds – rice, buckwheat, quinoa, chia seeds and, flax seeds

g.   All dairy products

h.   Water and, non caffeinated beverages

T4 to T3 conversion

Generally thyroid function is analyzed by TSH values. The pituitary gland in your brain release TSH which tells your thyroid gland to make T4. However your body must convert T4 into T3 (the active form) in order to use it If this conversion is poor then you may experience some of the common hypothyroid symptoms like fatigue, depression, weight gain, sensitivity, dig=fficulty concentrating and, more. So it is important to asses the conversion to find the root cause of the symptoms and, optimize thyroid function. There are many factors that influence this conversion stress, impaired liver function, poor intestinal health, low calorie diets.

So along with the thyroid function test you should also get the stress hormone, liver functioning and, GUT health parameters also checked. If found disturbed please check in the respective section of this chapter for special considerations.

Here I would like to mention that we need to take care of the below mentioned nutrients so that the T4 to T3 conversion is effective and, also the thyroid functioning is improved

Vitamin A, D, E, K

Zinc

Selenium

Iodine

Tryosine

Supplements for all these are available in the market.

4. Insulin Resistance

In this case the test done are

Fasting Insulin - should be less than 5

Fasting blood glucose - between 70 to 100

HBA1C - less than 5.7%

Leptin – less than 5

If these above mentioned tests are not normal that means you are having insulin resistance which increases your risk for progressing to type 2 diabetes. Also if these tests are abnormal in any am=manner you are actually in a pre-diabetic stage.

This increases the risk of being over weight especially belly fat, having high triglycerides and, also having elevated blood pressure.

When you have insulin resistance your pancreas makes extra insulin to make up for it. For a while this will work and, your blood sugar will stay normal. Overtime, though, your pancreas won't be able to make up. If you don't make changes in the way you eat and, exercise, your blood sugar levels will rise until you have prediabetes and, finally diabetes.

This problem if not handled with care will definitely disturb your body transformation goals.

Work out Considerations

Regular exercise is one of the best ways to increase insulin sensitivity. It helps move sugar into the muscles for storage and, promote an immediate increase in insulin sensitivity which lasts upto 48 hours. AS per studies both aerobic and, resistance training increases insulin sensitivity, combining both in your routine appears to be most effective.

There are some other specific advantages in such cases

a. Regular exercise can Improve overall and, disease specific quality of life.

b. Regular activity will enhance and, improve insulin sensitivity

c. Exercise contributes to an increased metabolism, which will help in weight management.

d. It will lower blood pressure, triglycerides and, resting heart rate

e. Increases efficiency for maintaining normal blood glucose with time

Diet Considerations

Let me tell you very clearly that this is a pre diabetic stage, no matter how much you cut down your calories and, work out for several hours, still your body transformation goals will be far off.

Importantly, eating the wrong foods can raise your blood sugar with insulin levels and, promote inflammation. Wit in no time if not controlled this pre diabetic stage will turn into a diabetic stage and, you will not be aware also.

It is important to understand the term Glycemic index

Carbohydrate is an essential part of our diets, but not all carbohydrates are equal. The glycemic index is a relative ranking of carbohydrate in foods according to how they affect blood glucose.

Carbohydrates with a low GI value that is 55 or less are slowly digested, absorbed and, metabolized and, cause a lower and, slower rise in blood glucose and, therefore insulin levels.

There are three classifications

Low – 55 or less

Medium – 56-69

High 70+

The table for glycemic index of foods is given in the mean planning chapter.

Research has proven that healthy low Glycemic index diet will be the only solution in case of insulin resistance, it helps to manage blood glucose levels, blood cholesterol levels and, gradually reduce insulin resistance, which is important to reduce the risk of long term diabetes related complications.

High GI foods provide a quick burst of energy where as low GI foods provide sustained longer lasting energy. Low GI foods are broken down slowly, trickling glucose into our system over a period of time. On the other hand, high GI foods cause a sudden spike in our blood glucose.

Here I would like to brief the entire scenario, in this case the problem is insulin resistance, that means body's cells are not accepting the insulin produced and, hence the unused blood glucose is converted into triglycerides and, then into fat. Now when we consume the high GI foods they immediately triggers blood glucose and, because of insulin resistance, more and, more is stored in terms of fat.

But on the contrary if we intake low GI foods, they will deliver blood glucose in stable manner and, the probability of triglyceride formation becomes less.

One more thing, the so called light food (that means high GI which are easily metabolized and, consumed by the body) which is termed good for weight management in normal case will be harmful for the person having insulin resistance. In this case it is better to consume food which is slowly metabolized. Surprising but true.

Foods to avoid – Your main goal should include staying away from unhealthy fats, liquid sugars, processed grains and, foods that contain refined carbohydrates. You have to avoid foods that increase your blood sugar levels and, drive insulin resistance.

1. Sugar sweetened beverages

2. Trans fats

3. White bread, pasta and, rice, all kinds of high carb, processed foods

4. Fruit flavored yogurt

5. Sweetened breakfast cereals

6. Flavored coffee drinks

7. Honey and, maple syrup

8. Dried fruit

9. Packaged snack foods

10. Fruit juice

11. French fries

12. Most fruits except berries

13. Cakes, cookies, pies, ice creams

Foods to eat – The main goal is to keep blood sugar levels well-controlled

1. Fatty fish

2. Leafy greens

3. Cinnamom

4. Eggs

5. Chia seeds

6. Turmeric

7. Greek yogurt

8. Nuts

9. Broccoli

10. Extra virgin olive oil

11. Flaxseeds

12. Apple cider vinegar

13. Strawberries

14. Garlic

In this case, reducing your carb intake may be beneficial. Studies have shown that a daily carb intake of 20-150 grams, or 5% – 35% of calories, not only leads to better blood sugar control but may also promote weight loss and, other health improvements. However, different individuals have different tolerance. Testing your blood sugar and, paying attention to how you feel at different carb intakes can help you find your range for optimal control, energy levels and, quality of life.

Following this approach can lead you towards your body transformation goals

Supplements available in the market

Many supplements may help to reduce insulin resistance. Keep in mind that you may experience different results based on factors such as duration supplement quality and, your individual status.

The supplements are

1. Cinnamon – Taken with meals
2. Ginseng – around main meals
3. Probiotics
4. Aloe vera
5. Berberine
6. Vitamin D
7. Gymnema sylvestre – a herb
8. Magnesium
9. Alpha lipoic acid
10. Chromium

5. Liver Functioning

Test to be done – AST and, ALT with other parameters

Reference values are as under

Before starting this subject we need to understand a term

"Non Alcoholic fatty liver disease"

It refers to a wide spectrum of liver diseases ranging from the most common, fatty lever that is accumulation of fat in liver to fat in the lever causing inflammation, then further to advance scaring of liver as a result of chronic inflammation.

All of the stages of non alcoholic fatty liver disease are now believed to be due to insulin resistance, a condition closely associated with obesity. In fact the body mass index correlates with the degree of liver damage, the greater the BMI the grater is the damage. The term non alcoholic is used because liver disease due to alcohol can show the same spectrum of liver disease. As expected, nonalcoholic fatty lever disease is now a days commonly observed. A sedentary lifestyle and, high calorie sugar and, fat intake lead to a high prevalence of obesity, insulin resistance, and, diabetes.

In most cases this disease causes no symptoms. It is discovered when routine blood tests show elevated levels of liver enzymes AST and, ALT in the blood.

Another way in which it is discovered is when ultrasound examination of the abdomen is done for other purposes, say for looking for gall bladder stones, and, fat is found in the liver.

In later stages of this disease it can lead to liver failure, swelling of the legs, accumulation of fluid in abdomen, bleeding from the veins and, mental confusion.

From the body transformation point of view if the AST and, ALT are more than 20, you definitely need to take care of your liver aspects.

Work out considerations

1. More of endurance work out should be practiced so that target heart can be achieved and, maintained for a long period of time to burn more and, more fat.

2. High-intensity interval training will certainly be a big support and, should be done atleast twice a week.

3. Muscle weakness is a side effect in this case, so strength training should be seriously done.

Diet Considerations

1. All the saturated fats and, trans fat should not be consumed.

2. Only monounsaturated fats like olive, peanut and, canola oils, Polyunsaturated fats which are found in greatest amounts in corn, soybean and, safflower oils and, many type of nuts.

3. Omega 3 fatty acids should be consumed which are found in oily fish like salmon, walnuts and, flaxseed oils.

4. Eat more low Glycemic index foods such as fruits, vegetables and, whole grains. These foods affect blood glucose less than high Glycemic foods like white bread, white rice, potatoes etc.

5. Avoid foods and, drinks that contain large amount of simple sugars, like soft drinks, sports drinks, sweetened tea and, juices.

6. Avoid alcohol use, it can further damage your lever.

Supplements available in the market

1. Milk Thistle

2. N-acetylcysteine

3. Artichoke leaf

4. Turmeric root

5. Dandelion root

6. Beetroot

7. Ginger

8. Choline

9. Molybdenum

10. Selenium

6. Uric acid

Uric acid reference values are as follows:

Uric acid is a waste product made by the body when it digest certain foods. When uric acids levels are high, crystals of it can accumulate in your joints. This process triggers swelling, inflammation and, intense pain. Most people who have the condition experience these symptoms because their bodies cannot remove the excess uric acid efficiently. This lets uric acid accumulate, crystallize and, settle in the joints.

Here I would mention high blood concentrations of uric acid leads to gout, diabetes and, kidney stones.

Work out Considerations

As it is clear from the above discussion, that in case of high concentration of uric acid, joint inflammation and, pain is a big issue. In that case it is not easy continuing smoothly with the work outs. The work out considerations will be same as in ESR and, CRP levels as the consequences relating to joints is the same.

In this case there are three levels of exercises

Level 1 - Therapeutic exercises, prescribed by health professionals, address specific joints or body parts affected by the joint pains. A therapeutic exercise program is often a necessary first step for individuals who have been inactive, have restricted joint motion or muscle strength.

Level 2 - If you have never really exercised before or have a condition that keeps you away from doing rigorous activity go for a lighter work out that last for atleast 30 minutes. Even Moving a little bit each day will bring down the inflammation.

Like you can go for a walk at a brisk pace

a. Stretching daily can help reduce stiffness and, increase range of motion.

g. Flowing movements like yoga, gentle poses or meditation can help

h. Water exercises – water helps support bodyweight, that means that water exercises do not impact heavily on the joints. Water treadmills are also available now a days.

i. Cycling – stationary or outdoors can be a safe way to get the joints moving and, improve cardiovascular fitness

j.   Strength training with a resistance band and, light weights will help to strengthen muscles around the joints, it will support the joints.

Level 3 – Starting a regular exercise program can be very challenging. You should be very cautious about the selection of the exercises that are safe and, customized to your specific needs and, also you have to monitor your body's response to exercise, and, modify your exercise routine as needed. Also you can make an exercise program in which you can primarily use the joints which are not paining or are less stiff and, give rest to the joints which are not that supportive.

Some guidelines are as follows:

f.   Set realistic and, short and, long term goals, and, reward yourself when you achieve them.

g.   Exercise with a partner or a professional

h.   Keep an exercise diary and, track your progress

i.   Identify problems or obstacles that are likely to trouble and, plan ahead to deal them

j.   Choose activities that are convenient, relatively inexpensive and, fun.

What not to eat

1.   All organ meats include liver, kidney and, brain

2.   Yeasts: Nutritional yeast, brewer's yeast and, other yeast supplements

3.   Asparagus, spinach, beans, peas, lentils, oatmeals, cauliflower and, mushrooms

4.   Added sugars – Honey and, high fructose corn syrup

5.   Sugary beverages especially fruit juices and, sugary foods.

6.   Refined carbs like white bread, cakes and, cookies

What to eat

1.   All fruits, cherries may help in lowering uric acid levels and, reduse inflammation

2. All vegetables are fine, potatoes, peas, mushrooms, eggplants and, dark leafy vegetables should be prioritize.

3. Lentils, beans, soybean and, tofu

4. All nuts and, seeds

5. Whole grains – oats, brown rice and, barley

6. Low fat dairy products will be beneficial

7. Eggs

8. Coffee, tea, green tea

9. All herbs and, spices

10. Plant based oils like canola, coconut, olive and, flax oils

7. Cortisol

Cortisol is a steroid hormone released by the adrenal glands. Whenever you experience something your body perceives as a threat, like a dog barking at you, a chemical known as ACTH (adrenocorticotropic hormone) is released in your brain. This triggers your adrenal glands to release cortisol and, adrenaline.

Test done

Reference ranges

Weight gain or loss is generally an issue both during and, after, times of increased stress. Increased stress levels tend to cause imbalance in cortisol, DHEA and, adrenaline. Cortisol in particular is often linked with weight fluctuation. Both an excess and, deficiency of cortisol can impact blood sugar levels, thyroid function and, metabolism. Signs of adrenal fatigue include low energy, trouble sleeping, frequent urination, weight gain, mood swings, depression, anxiety, brain fog and, auto immune disease.

There can be many aspects which disturbs cortisol levels like emotional imbalances, lack of sleep, excess sugar and, carbohydrate intake, irregular meals, severe infections, surgery or traumatic injury, excess endurance training, toxic exposures etc.

Work out Considerations

It is a fact that psychological changes have repeatedly been found to have real, measurable impact on our physical health. Especially stress, is a purely mental state but it triggers all kinds of physical changes in your bodies. These changes can affect virtually all the systems and, organs that are vital to our good health.

Staying fit can be great for your spirit and, physical health, but if you are suffering from severe or long term stress which leads to adrenal Fatigue, then you need to be very careful how you exercise. Here are some principles that you need to follow –

In case of initial levels of high cortisol levels and, adrenal fatigue

1. Vigorous exercises, any forms of endurance or strength training are permitted. During these stages your cortisol levels will tend to be high, vigorous exercise can actually help to moderate them.

2. You should try work out early in the day. This will keep your metabolism high. Exercising late in the day can interrupt sleep patterns which is already a problem in high cortisol levels

3. The length of your work outs should be inversely proportional to your age. Those who are younger will able to exercise for longer periods of time and, still remain fresh and, energetic. However with age metabolism slows down, extended work outs drain too much of our energy.

In case of later stages of high cortisol levels and, adrenal fatigue

1. In this case energy levels are extremely low, strenuous exercises should be avoided altogether.

2. Walking, swimming, yoga or similar low intensity work outs will boost the circulation without putting too much stress on your glands.

3. Short term high-intensity work outs will not be advisable, till you adapt yourself with regular training and, hard work.

Meditation and, deep breathing - I suggest that in this case Meditation should be considered as a must do work out and, it should be practiced regularly in your exercise schedule.

This technique enable to reduce stress and, normalize adrenaline and, cortisol levels. This allows the adrenal glands time for much needed regeneration. Also it improves circulation, eliminate toxins and, increase energy levels by increasing oxygen saturation. I assure that deep breathing and, meditation offers great valuable benefits.

Diet Considerations

1. A well balanced diet is the best way to keep your body healthy and, to regulate your sugar levels. It is recommended to have balanced protein, healthy fats and, high quality, nutrient dense carbohydrates.

2. Increase your vegetable intake to get the amount of vitamins and, minerals.

3. Include foods high in vitamin C, Vitamin B (especially B-5 and, B-6) and, magnesium to support healthy adrenal glands.

4. Timing your meals is really important. It helps with regulating blood sugar and, supporting adrenal glands.

5. Breakfast and, lunch should not be skipped, it forces your body to burn stored nutrients and, reduce your energy levels.

6. Eating regular, balanced meals and, healthy snacks, you can maintain your energy and, cortisol levels all day.

Food to eat

1. Lean meats
2. Fish
3. Eggs
4. Legumes
5. Nuts
6. Leafy greens and, colorfull vegetables

7. Whole grains

8. Dairy

9. Low sugar fruits

10. Sea salit in moderation

11. Healthy fats such as olive oil, coconut oil and, grapeseed oil

Foods to avoid

1. White sugar

2. White flour

3. Alcohol

4. Caffeine

5. Soda

6. Fried food

7. Processed food

8. Fast food

9. Artificial sweeteners.

Supplements available to improve Adrenaline health

1. Licorice root

2. Curcumin

3. Vitamin D

4. Phosphatidylserine

5. Rhodiola rosea

6. Ashwandha

7. Tryosine

8. Magnesium

9. Holy basil leaf

10. Vitamin C

Stress Levels are increasing day by day, in that case the Cortisol levels increases which disturbs our metabolism, immune system, blood pressure and, response to stress.

In all the above aspects, it is really difficult to continue with our body transformation goals. We need to get our cortisol levels checked and, take the nutrients and, diet accordingly.

8. Reproductive hormones

Tests to be done:

For men – Total Testosterone, Free Testosterone

For Female – Estrogen, progesterone, LH, FSH

Testosterone – Testosterone levels are higher in men, yet the hormone plays several vital roles in both – men and, women. One of its most important functions in both the genders is to maintain muscle mass and, promote muscle growth and, bone strength. Testosterone promotes muscle growth and, at the same time suppress fat gain also. Muscle burn far more calories than fat tissue. Lack of muscle thus puts people at a higher risk of eating too much and, storing the excess calories as fat.

obesity itself suppress testosterone. On average obese people have 30% testosterone levels than those who are normal weight.

a. First belly fat contains high levels of the enzyme aromatase, which converts testosterone into estrogen, the female sex hormone. This explains why obese men have higher estrogen levels than normal weight.

b. Second, high aromatase and, estrogen activity reduces the production of gonadotropin releasing hormone GRH, lack of which leads to low levels of luteinizing hormone which in turn reduce testosterone.

Estrogen – Estrogen is one of the two primary female sex hormones. It has many functions including

a.   Helping to control blood cholesterol levels

b.   Promoting bone health

c.   Protecting the brain and, mood

There are main three types of estrogen

a.   E1 – Estrone

b.   E2 – estradiol

c.   E3 - Estriol

Causes of estrogen imbalance may include PCOS, lactation, ovary removal, anorexia – eating disorder – not taking enough calories, vigorous exercise.

As discussed estrogen levels may be low because of many reasons. The most common reason is menopause. This is when a women's reproductive hormone decline and, menstruation stops. Many women notice that they gain weight this time in their life. One reason why people weight gain is changing hormone levels. One form of estrogen called estradiol decreases at menopause. This hormone helps to regulate metabolism and, bodyweight. Lower levels of estradiol may lead to weight gain. Throughout their life, women may notice weight gain around hips and, thighs. However after menopause, women tend to gain weight around their mid section and, abdomen. This type of fat gain tends to build up in the abdomen and, around the organs where it is known a s visceral fat and, it is dangerous and, it can lead to medical conditions like diabetes, stroke and, heart diseases

Diet Considerations in Testosterone imbalance:

A person's testosterone level will fall naturally with age by 1 to 2% per year, but some medical conditions, lifestyle choices and, other factors can influence the amount of this hormone in the body. A person can encourage the body by making some changes in diet and, lifestyle.

Testosterone boosting foods

1.   Ginger

2.   Oysters

3. Shellfish

4. Red meat

5. Poultry

6. Beans

7. Nuts

8. Pomegranates

9. Vitamin D Fortified foods

10. Leafy green vegetables

11. Fatty fish and, fish oil

12. Extra virgin olive oil

13. Onions

Foods to avoid

1. Processed foods – prepacked meals and, snacks – more of trans fat

2. Canned or plastic packaged foods

3. Alcohol

Also it can be increased by lifestyle changes like losing weight, exercising regularly, building muscle through resistance training, getting enough sleep, reducing stress.

Diet consideration in estrogen imbalance

What to eat

1. Flaxseeds

2. Soybeans

3. Dried fruits

4. Sesame seeds

5. Garlic

6. Peaches

7. Berries

8. Wheat bran

9. Tofu

10. Cruciferous vegetables – broccoli, Brussels sprouts and, cabbage

Work out considerations

People often turn to supplements and, medications to treat hormone related health issues like stress, depression, lack of sleep, weight gain and, mood swings. The most important key to balancing your hormones lie in boosting your physical activity. Exercise should be incorporatedin lifestyle to enhance the quality of life and, help regulate testosterone and, estrogen.

Physical activity, help boost testosterone. Here I would mention that the symptoms of menopause are in part driven by the imbalance and, decline of estrogen. One way to combat this is to exercise. Getting heart rate up for at least a half hour every day helps boost estrogen levels, which can help improve the menopause symptoms.

A balanced combination of strength training and, cardio work outs to maximize health benefits and, boost hormone levels. High-intensity and, compound exercises like squats, lunges, pull ups, pushups, burpees etc with minimum rest time in between.

The more intense a work out, the more these hormones are released.

Lift heavy to boost hormones and, do forced repetition

Lower body work outs helps in balancing hormones

Consistency is also key to retaining a steady flow of healthy hormones throughout your body.

If you are trying to boost testosterone avoid regular long time steady cardio work outs.

Herbs boosting estrogen

1. Alfaalfa

2. Black cohosh

3. False unicorn

4. Chaste tree

Supplements to boost Testosterone

1. D Aspartic Acid

2. Vitamin D

3. Tribulus Terrestris

4. Fenugreek

5. Ginger

6. DHEA

7. Zinc

8. AShwagandha

9. **Vitamins and, Minerals, the micro nutrients**

Vitamin and, mineral deficiencies are prevalent among overweight and, obese individuals, although it is not clear whether specific deficiencies are increasing the risk of greater adiposity and, obesity or whether increased obesity leads to specific micronutrient deficiencies or may be both. For example Vitamin D deficient obese children improved their vitamin D status following weight loss and, alo in contrast it is reported that increasing the intake of calcium rich foods helped in reducing obesity.

Overall, it is increasingly clear that micronutrient deficiencies need to be controlled if you are looking for body transformation

All the micro nutrients are necessary, primarily the following mentioned are directly linked with obesity. The following need to be tested –

Anti oxidants – Vitamin E, Vitamin C, beta carotene, selenium – are low in obese people absence of these increase leptin resistance, increasing the risk of obesity

Vitamin E and, C deficiency leads to abdominal fat deposition

In low vitamin E, HDL are more susceptible to oxidation

Total carotene deficiency leads to insulin resistance

Vitamin A deficiency lead to weight gain

Vitamin D3 defficiency highly prevalent among obese individuals

B complex vitamins – Thiamene, B6, B12 and, folic acid

Zinc deficiency effects body composition and, also inflammatory response

Low iron is reported in obese people

Low calcium intake is associated with increased fat mass

Diet Considerations

All these micro nutrients and, others too can be obtained by a balanced diet and, having all the possible foods for variety. Just understand all the foods available on the planet has some or the other nutrients. As per your convenience and, needs you should possibly eat all the foods.

Here are certain important micronutrients and, their sources

1. Water soluble vitamins –
    a. Vitamin B1 – helps convert nutrients to energy, source – whole grains, meat, fish
    b. Vitamin B2 – Necessary for energy production, cell function, fat metabolism, source – eggs, milk
    c. Vitamin B3 – Drives the production of energy from food, source – salmon, leafy greens, beans
    d. Vitamin B5 – Necessary for fatty acid synthesis, source – organ meats, mushroom, tuna, avocado
    e. Vitamin B6 – Helps body release sugar from stored carbs for energy, source- fish, milk, carrot, potatoe
    f. Vitamin B7 – help metabolizing fatty acids, amino acids and, glucose, source- eggs, almonds, spinach, sweet potatoe
    g. Vitamin B9 – Important for proper cell division, source – liver, black eyed peas, spinach, asparagus,
    h. Vitamin B12 – Necessary for RBC, proper nervous system and, brain function, source – fish, meat
    i. Vitamin C – pequired for the creation of neurotransmitters and, collagen, source – citrus fruits, bell peppers, Brussels sprouts

Fat soluble vitamins

a. vitaminA – Necessary for proper vision and, organ function, source – liver, dairy, fish

b. Vitamin D – Promotes proper immune function and, assist in calcium absorption and, bone growth, source – sunlight, fish oil, milk

c. Vitamin E – Assist immune function and, acts as an anti oxidant that protect cells from damage. Source – sunflower seeds, wheat germ, almonds

d. Vitamin K – Required for blood clotting and, proper bone developmentsource – leafy greens, soybean, pumpkin

Macro Minerals

a. Calcium – Necessary for proper structure and, function of bones and, teeth, assist in muscle function and, blood vessel contraction, source – milk products, leafy greens, broccoli

b. Phosphorus – Part of bone and, cell membrane source – salmon, yogurt, turkey

c. Magnesium – assist with over 300 enzyme reactions, including regulation of blood pressure – Almonds, cashews, black beans

d. Sodium – electrolyte that aids fluid balance and, maintenance of blood pressure, source – salt, processed foods, canned soup

e. Chloride – in combination with sodium, helps maintain fluid balance and, is used to make digestive juices, sources – salt, celery

f. Potassium – Electrlyte that maintain fluid status in cells and, help with nervous transmission and, muscle function, source – lentils, squash, bananas

g. Sulfur – Part of every living tissue and, contained in the amino acids methionine and, cysteine, source – garlic, onin. Brussels sprouts, eggs

Trace Minerals

a. Iron – helps provide oxygen to muscles and, assist in the creation of certain hormones, source – white beans, spinach

b. Manganese – assist in carbohydrates, amino acid and, cholesterol metabolism, source – Pineapple, pecans, peanuts

c. Copper – Required for connective tissue formation, as well as normal brain and, nervous system function source – liver, cashews

d. Zinc- Necessary for growth, immune function and, wound healing. Source – Chickpeas

e. Iodine – Assist in thyroid regulation- seaweed, cod, chickpeas

f. FLouride – Necessary for development of bones and, teeth, Source – fruite juice, water

g. Selenium – Important for thyroid health, reproduction and, defense against oxidative damage. – source – Barzil nuts, sardines

AS you can see all micronutrients are extremely important for the proper functioning of your body and, consuming an adequate amount, (I insist adequate amount, other wise it can be toxic also) of them is key to optimal health, fit body, and, may even help fight disease.

Nearly, supplements for all the micro nutrients are available separately in the market and, also as per their daily requirements certain multivitamins are also available in the market.

Micro Nutrients and, sudden weight gain – I have seen in some cases that when people start taking care of their micro nutrients there is a sudden weight gain and, they get tense, and, at time are really in a confused state, whether to continue with it or not.

Actually, you are ignoring the bigger picture. The moment you start consuming all the micro nutrients in right amount, our metabolism gradually start to function properly and, it leads to increase in some amount of muscle mass. That is the gain in good weight, infact you should be happy about it and, in larger perspective once it is settled, the increased metabolism will be effective in actual fat loss.

The second aspect is the appetite. Once we kick start our engine with all the necessary elements, our body demands right amount of calories, and, temporarily that may increase our appetite also, resulting in some weight gain. Don't worry that will settle down.

10. Food Allergies, Food sensitivities and, Toxicity:

Food allergies and, food sensitivities are often lumped together when it comes to the symptoms experienced after eating certain foods.

Food Sensitivities occur when the body is unable to digest certain compounds. Once the body ingests these foods, you experience those uncomfortable symptoms.

A food allergy, on the other hand is an immunologic response. Ehen you eat something you are allergic, your immune sustem negatively responds to the allergen. To protect the body, immune system tries to fight the allergen by unleashing natural bio chemicals that cause the allergic reaction you experience.

In this case Inflammation is the culprit. Inflammation is one of the reactions that occurs when the immune system is triggered by food allergies.

As we have discussed above also chronic inflammation leads to weight gain and, definitely disturbs your body transformation program.

Symptoms of food allergies usually affect one or more of the following parts of the body

a. Skin – including hives, tingling, itching and, redness.

b. Digestive systems – including abdominal pain, metallic taste in the mouth, swelling or itching of the tongue.

c. Respiratory system – including coughing, wheezing, nasal congestion, trouble breathing and, tightness in the chest.

Test to be done

Food allergies and, food sensitivities tests – IgE antibodies in the bold

Common food allergies

a. Lactose, sugar found in milk or dairies

b. Gluten, the main protein found in wheat and, few other grains

c. Fructose, the primary sugar in fruit juice, honey, sodas and, other beverages containing high fructose syrup and, alcohol

    d. Corn

    e. Eggs

    f. Soy

    g. Peanuts

    h. Nuts

Diet considerations

Food allergies and, reactions can be confusing. Often, it's not easy to figure out which foods contain ingredients that may trigger a reaction. Further, many people who think they are allergic to a food may actually be confusing a food reaction for an allergy and, may not need to eliminate certain foods.

At this time, there are no medications that cure food allergies. The most important treatment is the elimination of the allergy-causing food. Careful reading of ingredient labels is essential to avoiding all foods with the allergy-causing ingredient. For example, milk may be listed by its components casein or whey, and, eggs can be labeled as albumin. If you have an allergy to a certain food, you must become familiar with all related ingredients that could potentially cause a reaction. A good rule of thumb is, when in doubt, don't eat it.

Evolving research suggests that certain probiotics ("friendly" bacteria) may help to prevent or moderate the effects of some allergies.

Once you have identified all the possible medical and, internal complications, I won't say the body transformation journey will be easy but yes it will be smooth and, will give regular results and, also I insist, this testing is not a one time procedure.

In first attempt you will identify all the possible risk factors, gradually steps will be taken and, with time after 30 to 45 days you will get the problematic aspects tested again and, look for the improvement. If there are some improvements then get along with the precautions you are taking and, if there is no improvement then you need to re calculate all the possibilities and, all the remedies and, start working on it more seriously.

Till you get rid of all these complications, it will never be easy for you to achieve your targets in the desired time frame.

My last words in this chapter is, I have seen many cases who give up after certain time, just because, either they are not aware of the internal complications or knowingly they do not work on them and, try to just increase their work outs to the maximum or at the most follow some diet.

As I always say body transformation cannot be only achieved by working hard, you need to work smart also.

Please take care

CHAPTER 8

INJURIES AND, WORK OUT

Obesity and, pain

It is really difficult to figure out that the physical discomfort or in easy language, the pain, it can be

a. Knee pain

b. Low back pain

c. Shoulder pain

d. Ankle pain

e. Wrist pain

f. Elbow pain

g. Neck pain

h. Pain in hip joints

i. headache

Or anywhere in body. The medical term would be musculoskeletal pain.

Rather than finding a strong treatment for pain or exact cause of the pain, either we ignore it, or at times put some ointment, or do some popular home remedies or at the last when we don't see any solution we start taking medications like pain killers to suppress it for the time being. Do we ever try to think why this pain is there, or how come this pain started one day and, now it is getting on your nerves making you restless, why?

Trust me, the pain is a sign, your body want to tell you something. Just imagine a new born baby, whenever there is trouble he starts crying, now you have to figure out, what is the issue. Similarly the body signals through that pain, now find it out and, cure it or as time passes, the under lying cause of that pain will be increasing and, it will turn into a disaster and, also a day will come when it will effect the entire system internally and, externally.

Look, if chronic pain starts or persist after any kind of injury or an accident, then the case is different but otherwise if you have pain in your body then, there can be certain reasons

a. Obesity, due to excess pressure on joints and, tissues

b. Muscle weakness, it can be due to many reasons

c. Some medical issues like arthritis, thyroid imbalance, neuromuscular disorders, auto immune diseases, inflammation etc

d. It can be due to improper diet or deficiency of certain macro or micro nutrients

e. It can be due to certain medications

f. Some complication at the time of birth

g. Alcohol in excess can also be a reason

It is really important to figure out, what is the reason, it can be done by one or more tests like

a. MRI or CT scan to examine the inner structures of the body

b. Nerve tests for nerve functioning

c. Blood tests to check for infections or other conditions or excess or deficiencies

Once you have figured out the cause of the pain, I would recommend to start the appropriate treatment.

Here are some of the treatment options

a. Physical therapy – where you can do the exercises to improve the quality of life.

b. Occupational therapy – where recommended exercises can be done to address weakness in any particular part of the body

c. Medications

d. Dietary changes

e. Surgery if required

Many a times I have seen that initially people ignore this pain, there may be many reasons for that, one reason I have understood with time is, that health is not the priority, we have many other priorities work, family, friends, society and, many other but body or health is kept to the last. Now see what happens, due to that pain we get less active or sedentary with time, gradually our metabolism gets weak and, other complications start. After a period of time trust me you will not be able to figure out that the pain is due to your health problems or health problems are because of that pain. A time will come when, knowingly you will want to but you will not be able to help yourself.

There is always a way out, we can definitely have thousands of options to work out by passing the pain, or keeping situation under control and, work out. Frankly speaking, 90% of people are doing it also.

I do not prefer that way as

Firstly, the challenge is to be fit and, not to just look fit, removing or reducing the pain or I would say completely eradicate the reason of the pain, will considered to be a true victory.

Secondly, with the pain it will be at times difficult for us to work out regularly, the work out variations will be limited and, the intensity of the work out will have to be kept controlled.

So it is better not avoid, and, find the root cause of that pain and, take necessary action immediately and, on the other hand start the body transformation process with corrective measures.

The day when you think about body transformation, as we started, first step is assessment, pain, it's causes and, it's treatment is also part of the assessment. It is really important to figure out all the aspects regarding pain. Pain free work outs are always better than work out with pain.

Seven rules to deal with all kinds of pain and, continue with the targets

Do not worry if you have an injury, you can still work out and, achieve your goals, you just need to be determined and, be calculated about your every move.

In my exercising career of around 30 years, I have struggled with many injuries, still tried to carry on with my work outs on daily basis. Following rules are, what I follow, and, I will share with you—

1. ***You will be your own judge*** – When you are in pain, everyone around you will ask you to stop. It is only your willpower that will stand by you. You have to decide whether you wish to fulfill your goals or let the situation worsen further. I warn you that the external motivation will be absolute zero when you begin. You have to believe in yourself and, progress slowly but steadily, without aggravating your injury or pain. You have to work out strictly in a progressive manner by keeping all the safety measures in mind and, pushing yourself by only a 0.0001% every day. Depending on the severity of your injury or pain, only you can decide to either progress, maintain or stop. For example we have a shoulder pain, that too severe, in this case you are not able to do pushup or bench press or shoulder presses or some exercises. You can start the exercises with minimum weight. If you want to do pushups you can do knee pushups or simply just hold on to a plank. Just understand, in the area of pain, you need to maintain blood circulation so that all the nutrient circulation is there and, the injured area recovers otherwise the situation will get worse. As I always say, it's like a terrorist attack in certain part of the country, what government officials will do, it will send forces in that area, to control things. If the forces are not sent, the situation with time will be out of control and, get worsen. Similarly in body where there is injury or pain we need to maintain blood circulation and, it will be maintained if we work out and, that too with only 1% intensity in beginning and, then as it gets stronger and, better you can increase the intensity.

2. ***Only one tire is punctured at a time*** – In a car generally one tire is punctured at a time, rest are working. I have seen that people in case of pain or an injury in any body part, they stop the entire work out. This is not the right way. If a certain joint or muscle is not functioning 100%, we can definitely keep it resting and, continue with our work out. Like if lower body is in pain like in case of some knee or ankle injury we can definitely have alternate exercises to work the surroundings or we can work out the upper body for meanwhile. This will keep us in motion and, help in maintaining our fitness.

3. ***Body has its own repair system or reflex mechanism*** – Technically speaking – in case of a muscle, bone, ligament or tendon injury, minor or major, there is body's natural defense. Research has shown that "The healing response is generated by the living parts of the bone, the cells that live within the matrix". Healing faster is not any magic. When we say matrix, we are talking about the light weight but during calcium carbonate structure makes up most of your bone. Inside little pockets in the matrix are living cells, including bone building osteocytes. When you break a bone, they are released from the pockets. Don't take it lying down. A busted bone, or some muscle or bone injury is not a six month excuse to keep sitting idle without any work out. You have to introduce a modicum of stress on the bone to stimulate those osteocytes to lay down more bone. Most breakdowns are ready for light stress after six weeks. Then you can gradually increase the intensity progressively.

4. ***RICE principle*** – it works

   REST – Give rest to the injured area

   ICE – Put cold packs or ice packs

   Compress – Tighten it up with a wrap or bandage

   Elevate – Elevate the area for reverse blood flow.

   This principle definitely works in any kind of acute injury.

   In case of chronic pain, you may put heat pads and, let it relax. You can also take massages and, physiotherapy is also a great treatment.

5. ***Proper nutrition is important*** – Some change in diet can reduce pain and, help you to recover faster.

    a)   Take foods rich in protein – Firstly body's pain relivers are derived from protein which is Amino Acids and, they make their way into the blood stream through the intestine. They then act as building blocks for compounds that help with pain reliefs.

         Secondly muscle cartilages needs protein to grow.

         Thirdly protein helps in activation of glucagone which increases blood glucose levels and, blocks glucose storage as fat. This prevents arise in insulin levels, carbohydrate cravings and, relieves pain.

         Lastly protein helps in decreasing inflammation as certain protein rich foods contain anti inflammatory properties, lowering experience of pain.

    b)   Keeping a balanced or calculated calorie intake – in case of injuri if weight increases, which definetly happens as you are not able to work out due to injury and, in addition to that if calories are also uncontrolled, it will lead to excess weight carried around weight and, obesity. Both of which make the pain worse, as it puts extra pressure on joints and, inflammation.

    c)   Avoiding foods which leads to inflammation – inflammation is a localized condition in which part of the body becomes redden and, painful in reaction to any injury or infection. There are cases when inflammation does not cease. In this case, many diseases, heath problems and, ultimately pain persist. Inflammation is discussed in the chapter of Special Population.

    d)   Increase the intake of Omega 3 fatty acids- Our bodies, unfortunately, don't produce Omega 3. It is an essential mineral. It has been proved that optimal doses of Omega

3 fatty acids can provide relief from pain. Also, it is anti-inflammatory. It is found in fish like salmon and, tuna, olive oil, some plants and, nuts.

e)   Making sure you take enough vitamins and, minerals. Some musculoskeletal problems are a result of vitamin deficiencies, if taken correctly, they can help soothe pain.

i)   Vitamin D: helps in calcium absorption.

ii)   Vitamin K: Plays a large part in cartilage metabolism and, is a promoter of cell survival, both of which are very important processes. We can obtain the said vitamin by consuming; green leafy veggies like Lettuce, Spinach and, Beans.

iii) Vitamin B: Helps in keeping the blood corpuscles and, neurons healthy and, aids in DNA formation, the genetic material present in our body cells.

iv) Calcium and, Phosphorus: These are bound together as a crystal-like mineral that is embedded into collagen that forms the framework of our body as we grow and, develop. The special combination of minerals and, proteins in bones gives them their strength and, rigidity. The recommended intake of calcium is 700mg daily for an adult. Proper doses of calcium will help in regenerating our cells in muscles.

6. ***Stretching and, passive work outs always work*** – In case of pains, you can continue to do stretching and, passive activities, which helps to maintain blood circulation. Here the intensity of the stretching should be controlled and, it should not increase the pain.

7. ***Active Rest*** – Last but not the least is the Rest. Some injuries and, pains take time, never get impatient or disheartened, give them time to heal. Take active rest, yes I wrote it correct "active rest". Be active in your daily routine and, carry on with the possible work outs and, give your injured area some rest and, time to heal.

Following all the above principles, with time, the injury will recover, pain will subside and, may be at a point the muscles or joints you must be feeling are the weakest will become your strongest areas.

How to deal with Lower back pain

Lower back pain is becoming a big issue with time. Most low back pain is the result of an injury, such as muscle sprains or strains due to sudden movements or poor body mechanics while lifting certain objects and, also due to lack of training or strengthening of the lower body and, core muscles.

Medically, low back pain can be the result of

a. Spinal cord cancer

b. Ruptured disc

c. Sciatica

d. Arthritis

e. Kidney infections

f. Spine infections

Acute back pain can last from a few days to few weeks, but chronic back pain may last longer. Here I would mention that the moment pain starts, general strategy is to safeguard that area, and, eventually which leads to improper blood flow in that area. In this case the muscles weakens, which makes the back more prone to injury.

You should seek medical attention immediately. Certain tests like X rays, CT scans, MRI and, ultrasounds may be necessary so your doctor can check for bone problems In bone, disc or ligaments and, tendons in your back. There are a number of possible medical treatments like medications and, medical appliances depending on the severity and, complexity of the problem.

Exercises to relieve Lower Back Pain:

Generally, people prefer to rest in case of the lower back pain, but it is actually recommended to keep exercising. Instead of running or heavy weight training, those suffering from pain can perform a few stretching exercises. It is always recommended to not go overboard and, stop when you are uncomfortable.

These exercises work by stretching out muscles that are abnormally tight when you have ache in your lower back and, strengthening the muscles that tend to be weak. Make sure that you do warm-up before you begin with stretching. You should never bounce during stretching and, all stretches should be slow and, gradual. Avoid over-stretching, stretch only until you feel a pop in your muscles. Hold every position for 20-30 seconds at least thrice if not five times. These are listed as follows:

❖ Abdominal Strengthening: Abdominal muscles are antagonistic to lower back, the Lower back pain always increases if and, when our abdominals are weak. If we strengthen our abdominals, our lower back would be relieved of some it's burden and, will be able to recover faster. Crunches (3 sets- 25 reps each), will help you achieve the said goal. You need to strengthen the transverse abdominis and, oblique muscles as they provide a lot of support to the lower back. The exercise for the same is twisted crunches. Lie down on the floor and, rest your legs in a 90 degree angle on a bench. Push yourself up to meet your thighs and, go back down. Repeat. (To be done thrice a week).

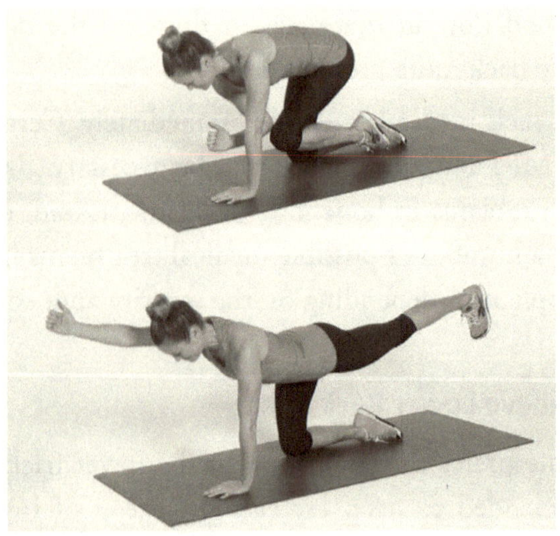

Bird-Dog crunches

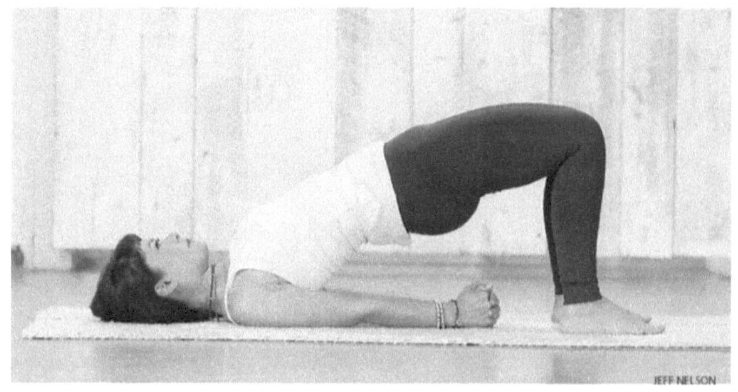

Bridge-pose

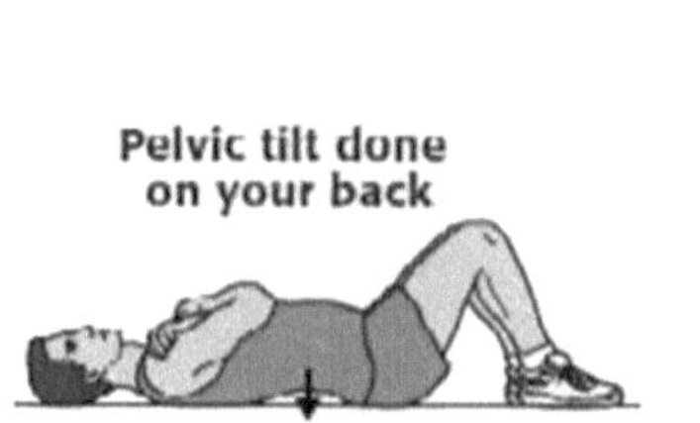

Pelvic tilt

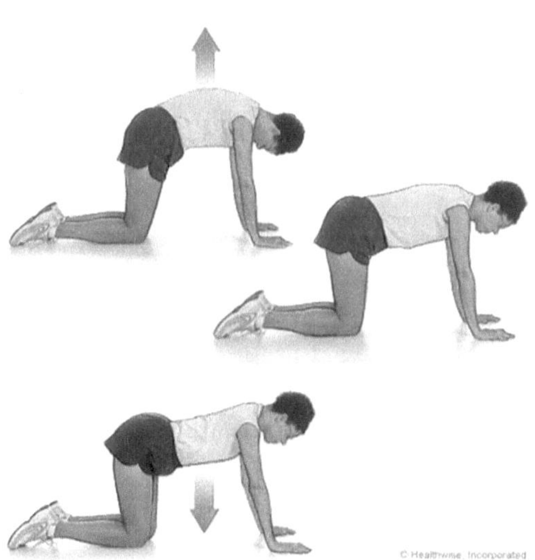

Cat and camel

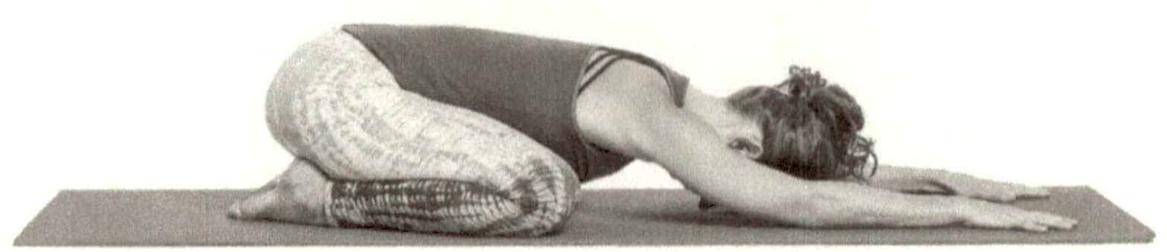

Child Poses

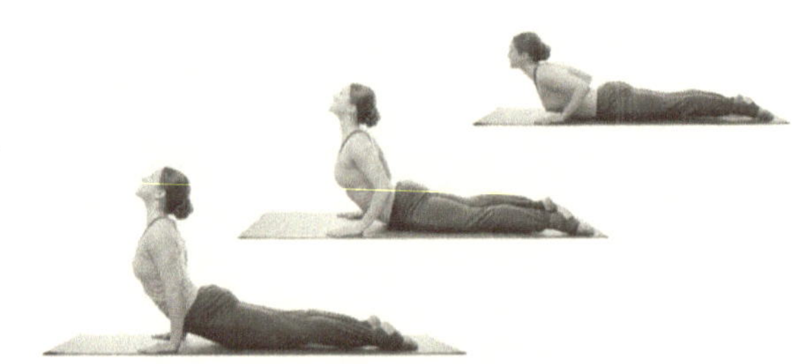

Cobra-pose

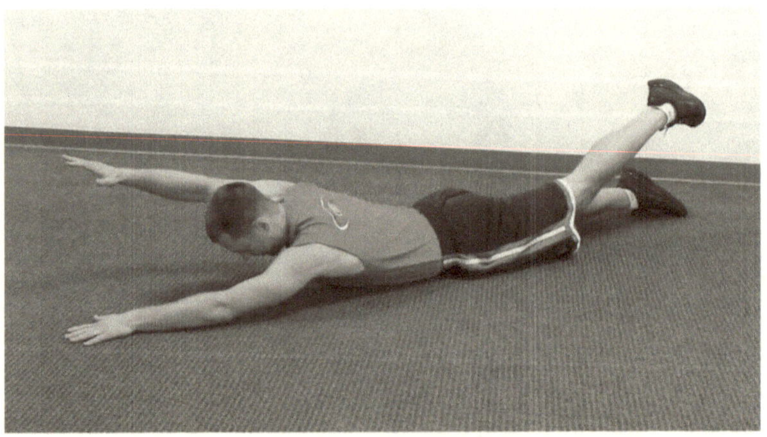

Lower Back align

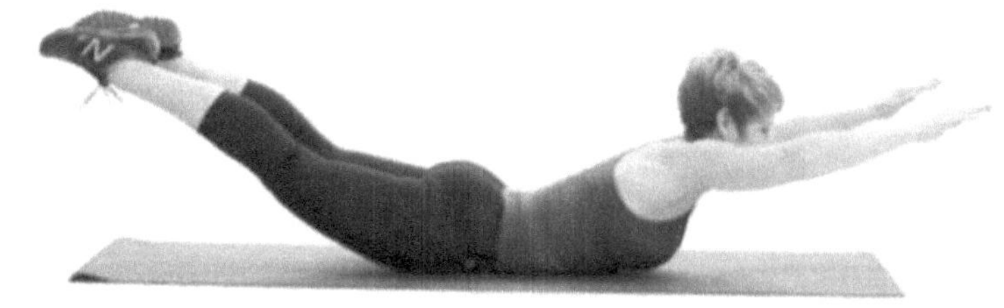

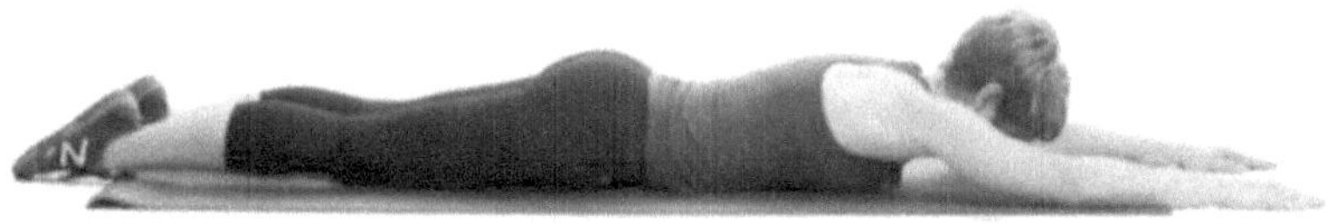

Hyper Extensions

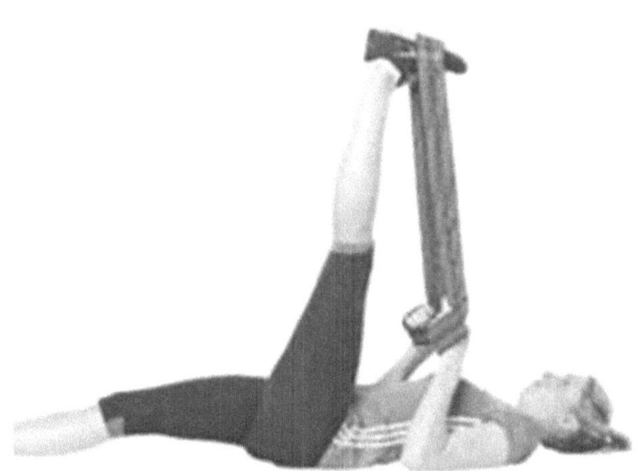

Halmstring stretch

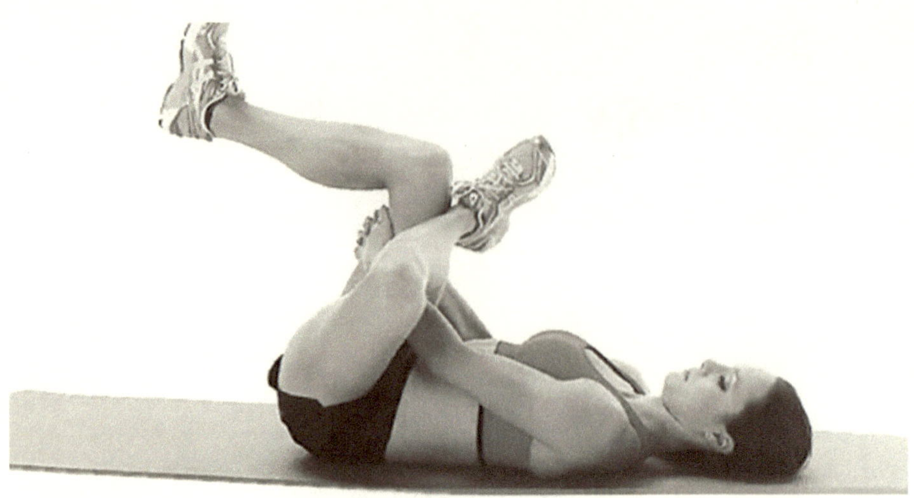

Piriformis stretch

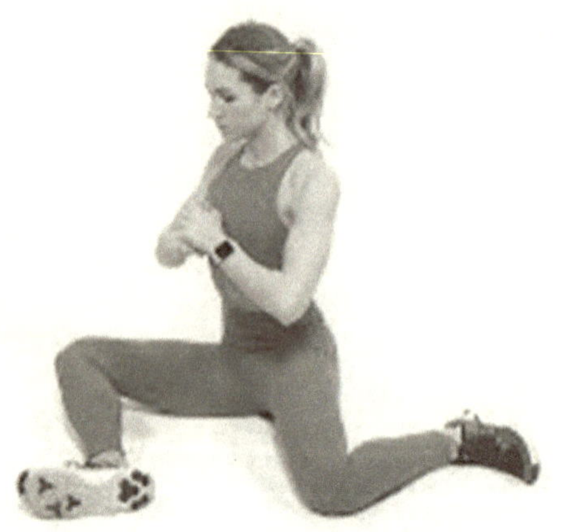

Hip stretch

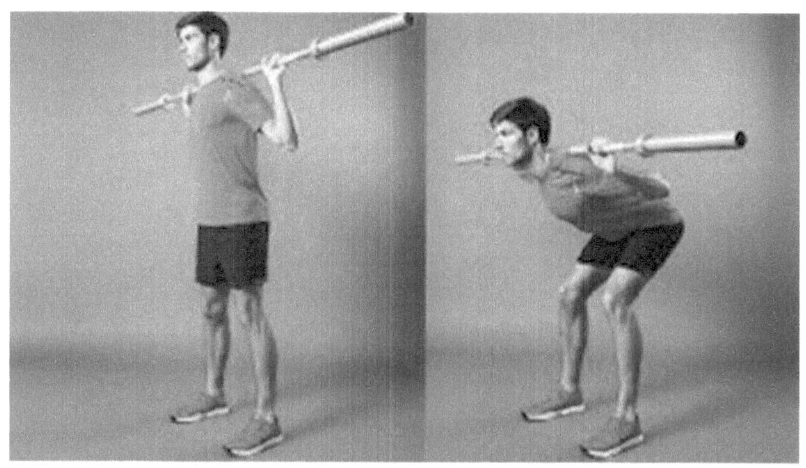

Good morning

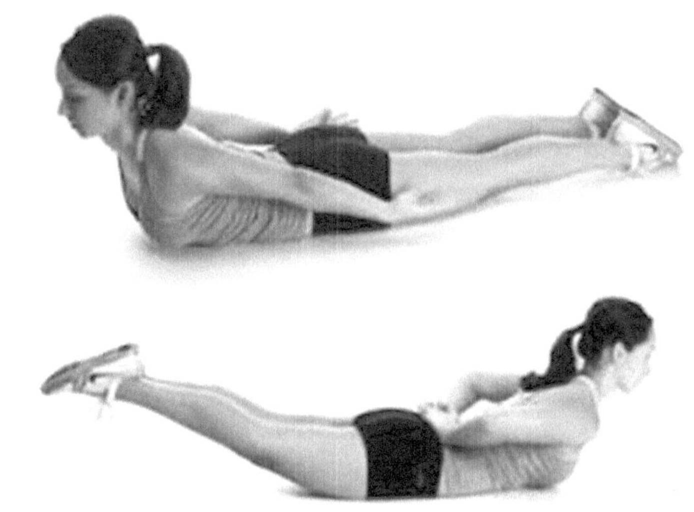

Hyper extensions

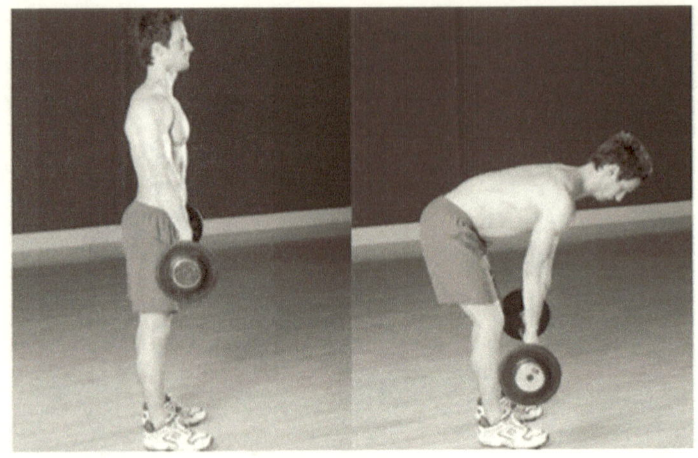

Stiff-leg-deadlift

* Bird Dog exercise

* Bridge Pose

* Pelvic Tilt

* Cat and, dog exercise

* Child Pose

* Cobra Pose

* Alternate hand and, leg up in supine position

* Both arms and, legs up

* Hamstring stretch

* Piriformis stretch

* Hip stretch

When you finally feel strength in your back, you can begin with,

* Good Morning

* Hyperextensions

* Stiff leg Deadlift

Begin without weights at first and, progressively train further.

Precautions when suffering from back pain:

* Avoid jumping, or jumps or bumps while travelling in a car or a two wheeler or any vehicle

- Postures should be taken care while sitting or standing. Stand erect on both knees soft, straight and, balanced and, never lean on one knee or against a wall, always walk or stand with abdominals tight and, lower back arched.

- If you have a sitting job or you have long driving hours, put back rest on to your seat for support and, correct posture.

- Avoid forward bending.

- Strictly do not lift anything from the floor with your knees straight and, bending forward, rather bend your knees and, then lift and, that too not really heavy.

- Practice the stretching and, back strengthening exercises mentioned at least thrice a week.

Precautions while work out

Avoid or be careful with the exercises like weighted squats, behind the neck shoulder presses, standing bicep curls, weighted dead lifts or lunges.

Avoid any exercise with weights while standing, do only in sitting with back supported or lying positions.

No forward bending exercises.

Prefer machines than free weights.

Avoid any kind of leg lift

Avoid full sit ups

Try wall sit for back strengthening

Walking, swimming or biking can be good options

Avoid running

Try yoga for core strength.

Important note – Our lower back is seated on our hips and, legs. In case these muscles are weak we can never strengthen our lower back. Do carefully strengthening exercises for lower body, with permitted range of motions and, without aggravating your pain.

Some suggestions are

Free bench squats – normal, close and, wide – all positions

Leg extensions in seated or lying positions

Leg curls in lying or seated positions.

Glute bridges.

Also you can select exercises from the strength section in the book for lower body training, which you are comfortable with.

Pain is nothing but, some weak muscles which need to be strengthened with training in a progressive mode.

How to deal with knee pain

Knee pain is a common complaint that affects people of all ages.

Symptoms may be Swelling, stiffness, redness, warmth to the touch, weakness, instability, popping or crunchy noise or inability to fully strengthen the knee.

Possible causes can be –

a) Injury – A knee injury can affect any of the ligament, tendons or fluid filled sacs that surround your knee joint as well as the bones, cartilage or ligament that form the joint itself. Injury can be ACL (anterior cruciate ligament) fracture, torn meniscus, knee burritis or patellar tendinits.

b) Mechanical problems – Hip or foot pain, dislocated knee cap or lose body.

c) Medical issues – Osteo arthritis, Rheumatoid arthritis, gout or septic arthritis, patella femoral pain which refers to pain rising between knee cap and, the thigh bone.

d) Excess weight – Being overweight or obese increase stress on your knee joints even during ordinary activities such as walking or climbing stairs. Also puts you to increased risk of osteo arthritis by accelerating the break down of joint cartilage.

e) Lack of muscle flexibility and, strength – Strong muscles around the knee joint helps to stabilize and, protect your joints, also muscle flexibility can help you achieve full range of motion.

f) Certain sports or occupation – Any daily requirement that emphasize repeated pounding your knees take when you run or jog or jump or do any other activity, all increase your risk of injury.

g) Any previous injury may re occur with the present activities that may inhibit your daily activities.

Whether you are an athlete or a daily walker, in case of knee pain it is always a problem to continue with your favorite activities. What ever may be the reason, stretching and, strengthening exercises may help ease the pain while improving your flexibility and, range of motion.

In addition to the seven rules given in the beginning of the chapter, the key is to strengthen and, activate the muscle groups surrounding the knee joint which are quad muscles, hamstring, shin bone and, calve muscles.

Remember whenever a joint is in a problem, the supporting muscles always play a major role.

Stretches

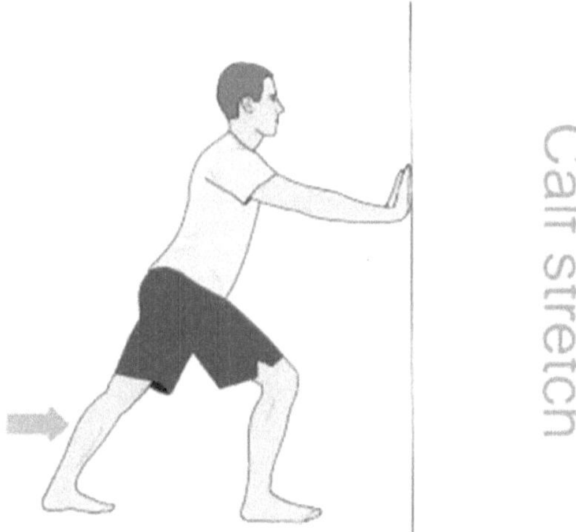

Knee and calf stretch

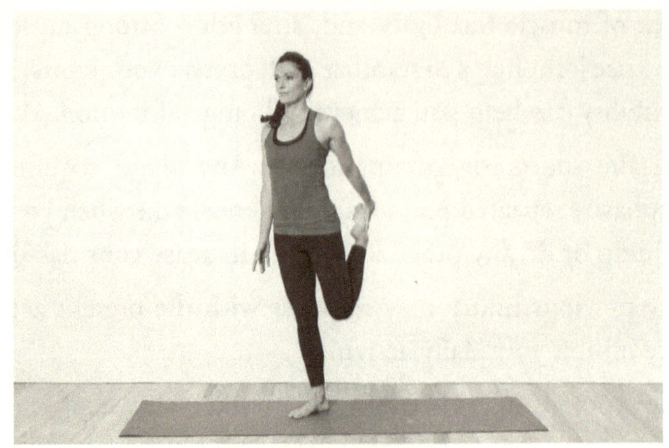

Quadricep stretch

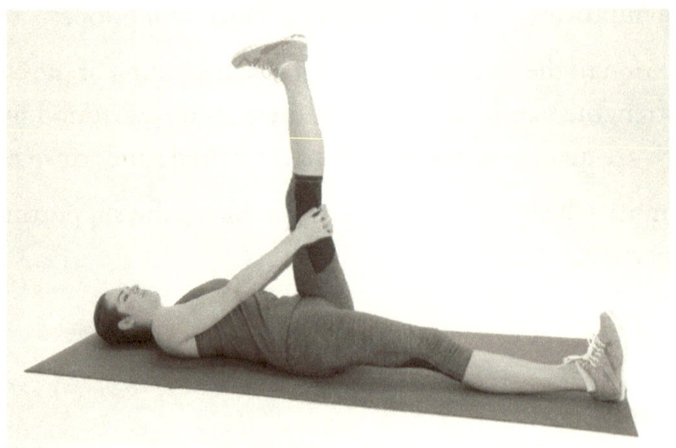

Hamstring-Stretch

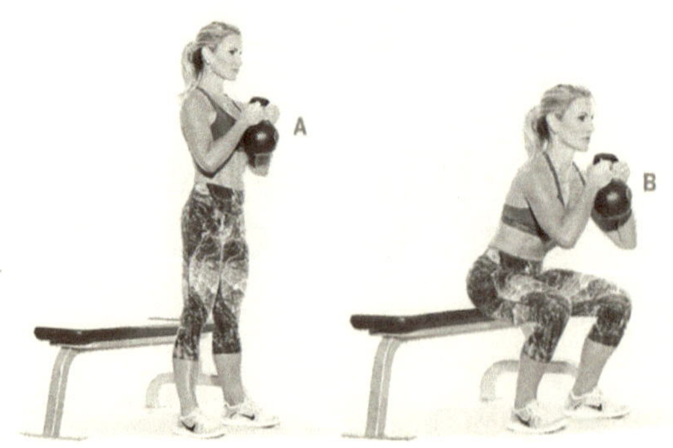

Bench squat

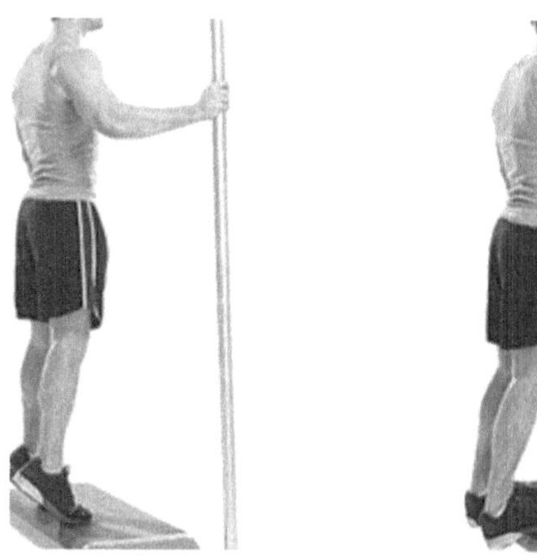

Calf raises

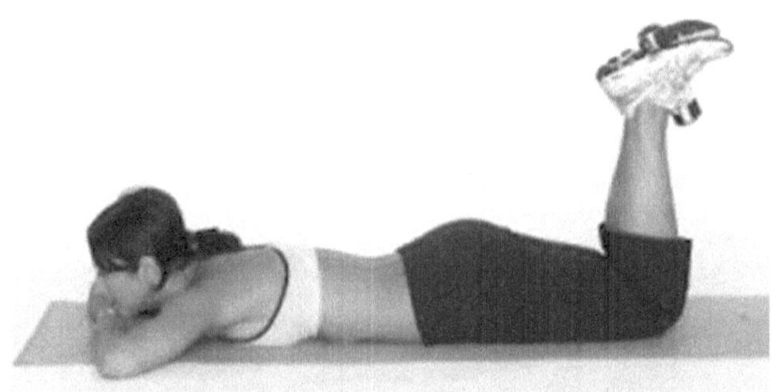

Halmstring curls

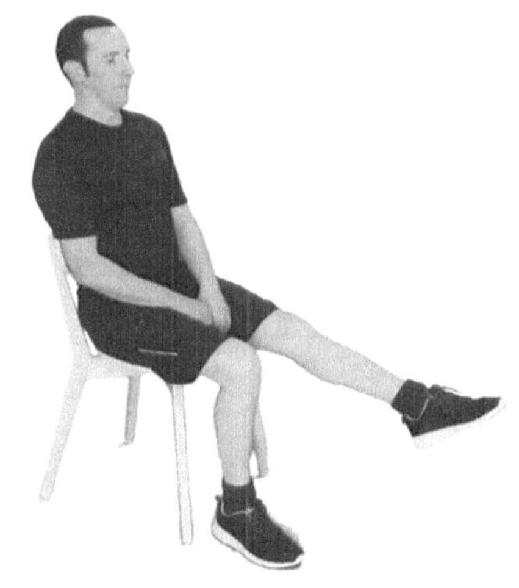

Leg extension

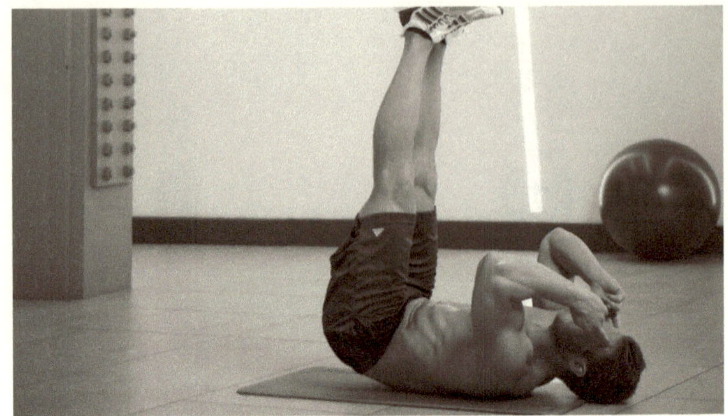

Leg-raise

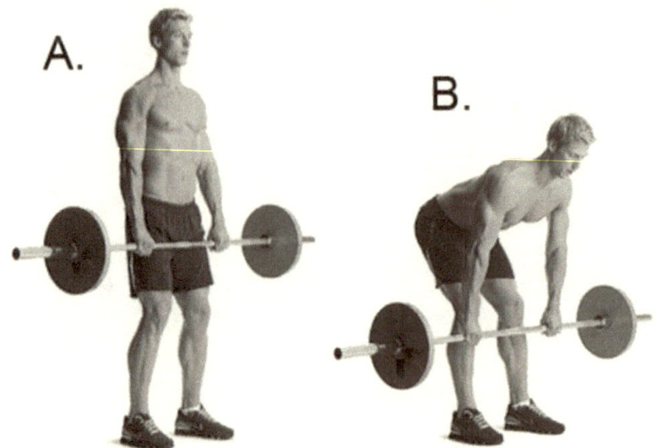

Stiff deadlift

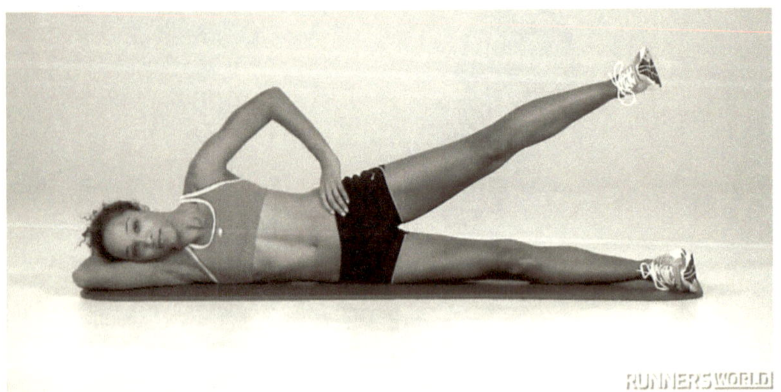

Side leg raises

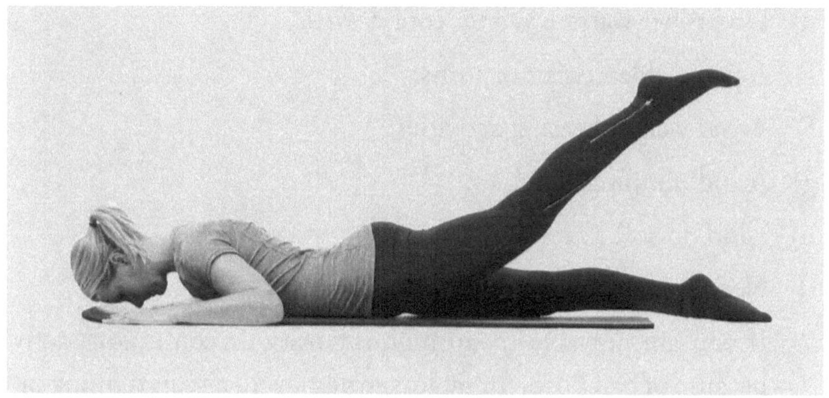

Prone leg raises

a)   Knee and, calf stretch

b)   Quadriceps stretch

c)   Hamstring stretch

Strengthening Exercises

a)   Bench Squat

b)   Calf raises

c)   Hamstring curl

d)   Leg extensions

e)   Leg raises

f)   Stiff leg dead lift

g)   Side leg raises

h)   Prone leg raises

Other exercises can be done when you have strengthened your muscles for some time like yoga, elliptical machine, swimming, cycling, water aerobics, walking etc.

Do's and, Don'ts

a)   Avoid running, outdoors or on treadmills.

b)   Avoid excess bending of the knee.

c)   Avoid squats or lunges, instead go for knee free work outs.

d) Do proper warm ups and, cool downs.

e) Avoid sudden twists or turns.

f) Avoid weight bearing activities.

g) Avoid jumping activities.

h) Land on soft knees.

i) Never ignore lower body work outs.

j) If you are not able to do high-intensity or continuous activities because of bad knees for fat loss, you may do circuit training or non stop work outs in order to burn more calories.

How to deal with shoulder pain

Shoulders, each, have two joints making it the most flexible part of the body. It is a ball and, socket joint. It is called as this because the top of the upper arm bone, the humerus, is shaped like a ball. This ball fits into the shoulder blade bone which acts as the socket, giving your shoulder a wide range of movement. This joint is very small, it's held together and, controlled by covering of the muscles, which are secured to the bones by strong chords called tendons. These muscles and, tendons form a capsule around the joint and, support its movement, but can make it more likely to dislocate than other joints.

Causes of shoulder pain –

a) Inflamation –

b) Damage to the muscles and, tendons around the shoulder.

c) Tension in the muscles between neck and, shoulder. Its often linked the way you sit, stand or work.

d) Arthritis

e) Neck problems – problem in neck can make shoulder blade or upper outer arm painful. It is known as reffered or raduated pain. Ifyou are feeling tingling sensation in arm or hand, as well as pain in shoulder, it's likely to be from a problem in neck.

Also shoulder pain can have causes that are not due to any disease, it can be due to overuse, disuse, sprain, strain or sleeping on side.

f) Swimmer's shoulder – caused by connective tissue rubbing on shoulder blade.

g) Rotators cuff tendnitis – swelling of the tissues connecting muscles and, bones in the shoulder.

h) Muscle strain - stretching or tearing of a muscle or tissue connecting to bone.

i) Rotator cuff tear – tear in the tissues connecting muscle to bone around shoulder joints.

Stretches

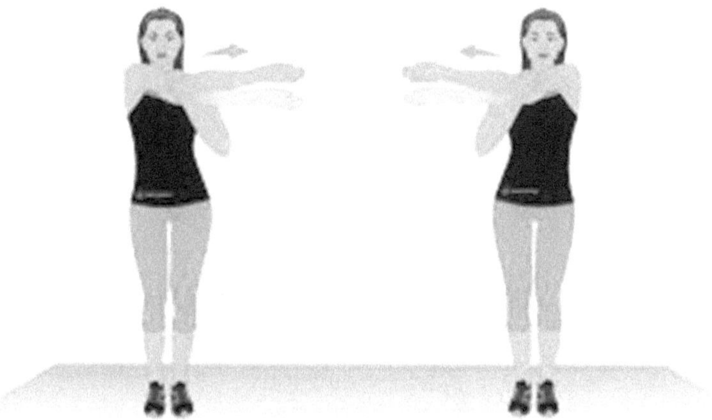

Across the chest stretch

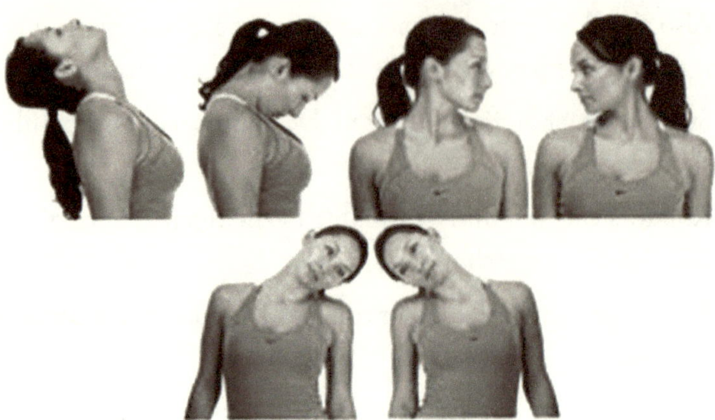

Neck rotate

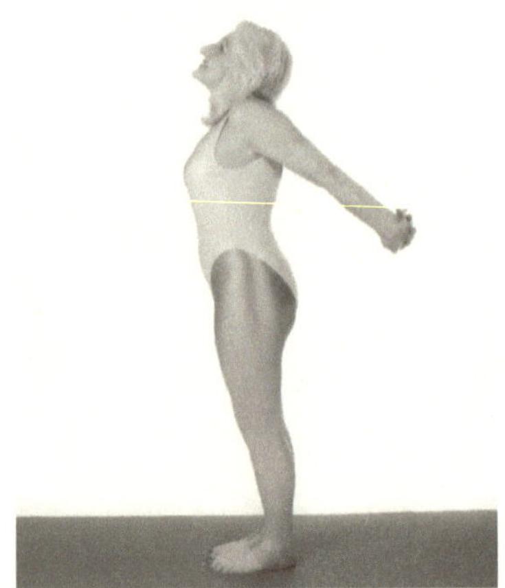

Chest expansion

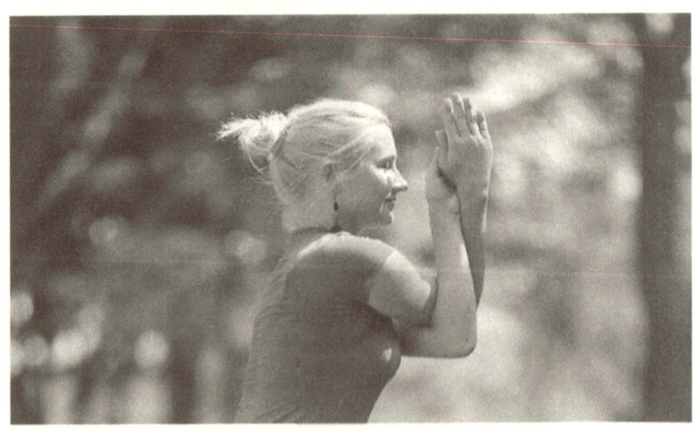

Eagle Arm

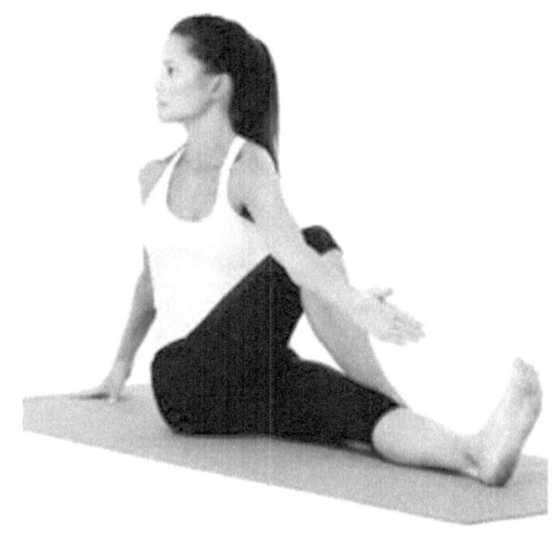

Seated twist

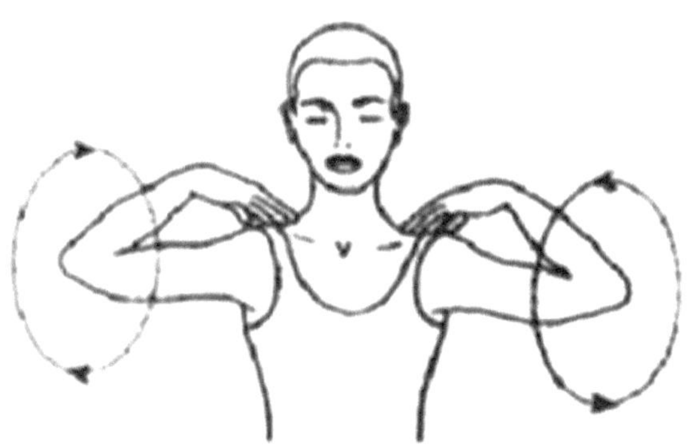

Shoulder circle

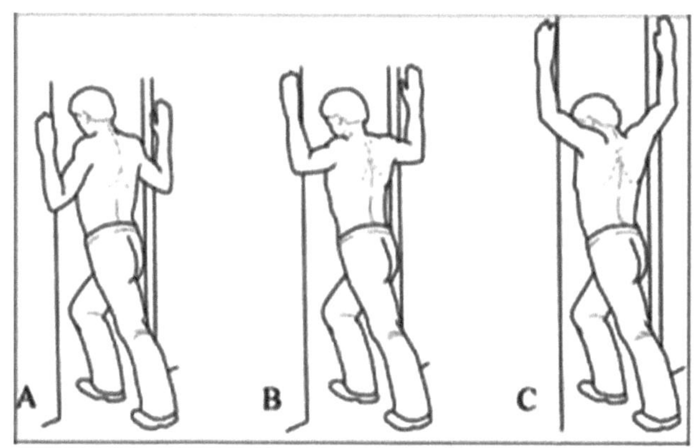

Doorway shoulder stretch

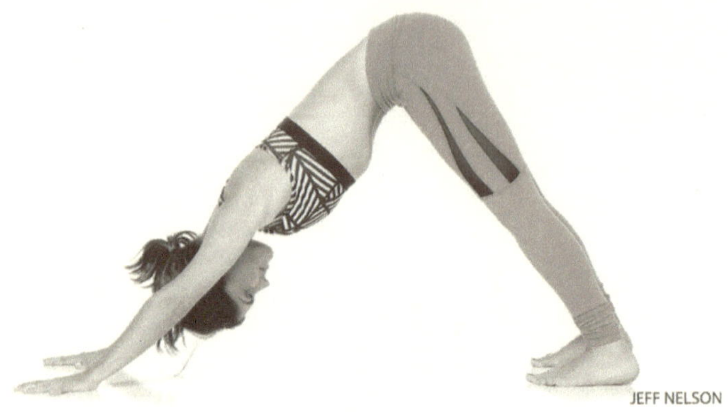

Downward-dog

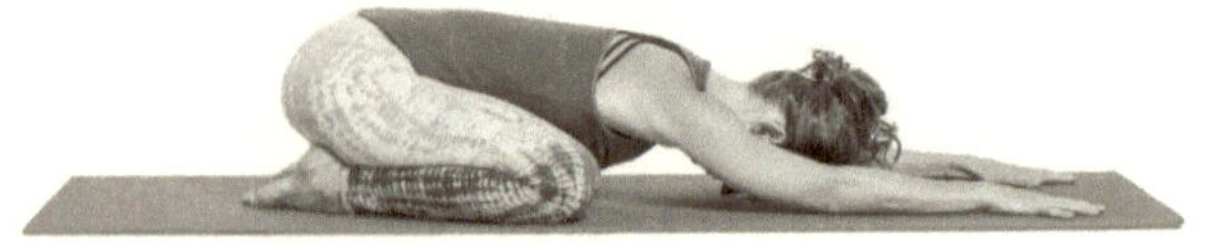

Childspose

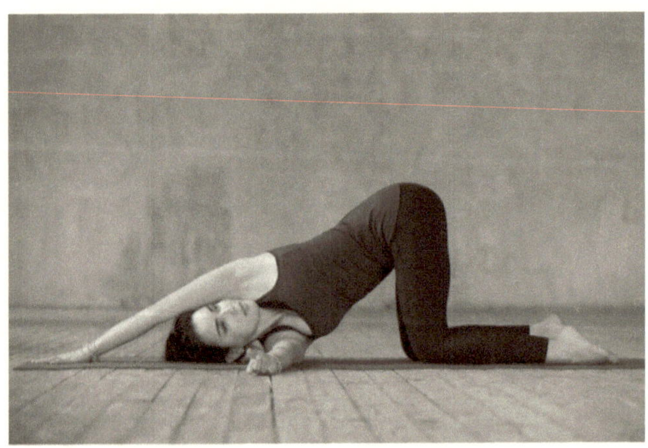

Thread-the-Needle-Pose

1. Across the chest stretch
2. Neck rotate
3. Chest expansion
4. Eagle arm spinal roll
5. Sitted twist
6. Shoulder circle
7. Door way shoulder stretch
8. Downward dog pose
9. Child pose
10. Thread the needle – all four, one arm twist under and, keep your head on floor and, other hand in hair

Follow all the 7 rules in shoulder pain also

Do's and, don'ts while work out

* Shoulder is the most worked muscle, may be its chest, or back bicep, or lower body. So warm up of shoulder muscle is really important before starting an work out.

* The care of shoulder pain – Avoid dumbbell behind the neck press, also do over the head movements in a controlled manner.

* Heavy pushing movements – should be avoided

* Heavy – deadlifts or other heavy liftings should be avoided

* Weight training should be progressively done.

How to deal with neck pain

Neck is made up of vertebrae that extend from the skull to the above torso. Cervical discs absorbs shocks between the bones. The bones ligaments and, muscles of your neck support your head and, allow motion

Neck pain and, stiffness can happen for a variety of reasons:

1. Muscle tension and, strain

a) Poor Posture

b) Working at a desk for too long without changing the position.

c) Sleeping in a bad or uncomfortable position.

d) Jerking your neck or keeping it stiff during exercises- known as whiplash.

2. Injury – The neck is vulnerable to injury especially in falls, sports or accidents, where the muscles and, ligaments of the neck are forced to move outside of their normal range. If neck bones (cervical vertebrae) are fractured, the spinal chord may also be damaged.

3. Meningitis – is an inflammation of the thin tissue that surrounds the brain and, spinal cord. In this case headache or fever often occur with stiff neck.

4. Rheumatoid Arthritis – It causes pain, swelling of joints and, bone spurs. When these occur in the neck area, neck pain can result.

5. Osteoporosis – weak bones can lead to some fractures, if in neck can lead to neck pain.

6. Age – With age cervical disc can degenerate, this is known as sondylosis or osteoarthritis of the neck.

Exercises to relieve Neck pain – A typical neck exercises program will consist of stretching and, strengthening exercises, aerobic conditioning and, possibly trigger point exercises.

Here I would like to mention, when neck, chest and, upper back muscles become tightened or elongated, the shoulder can become rounded and, the head sags forward. This poor posture in turn puts more pressure or stress on the cervical spine's facet joints and, inter vertebral discs as well as muscles and, ligaments.

Poor Postures with the head too far forward may lead to chronic neck pain and, can also be accompanied by stiff joints, upper back pain, shoulder blade pain and, headaches.

A Neck stretching and, strengthening program may help which is as follows:

Neck Stretching

a) Neck Extension – Gently extend the neck by looking upward and, bring the head backward while keeping shoulder and, back stationary, hold there and, gradually come back.

b) Neck flexion – Forward bending – Gradually lower the chin toward the chest and, look downward, hold and, gradually come back.

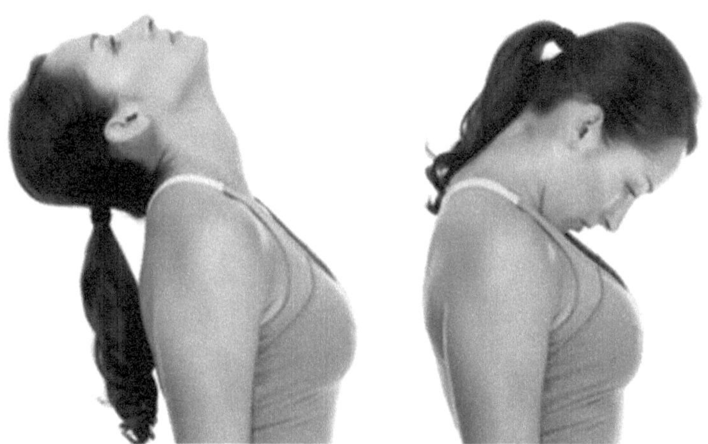

Neck_extension

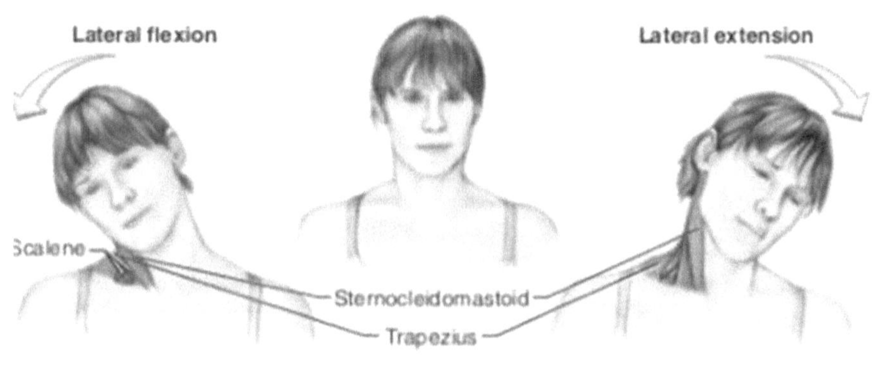

Lateral neck flexion

c) Lateral neck flexion – Bending side to side slowly and, gradually

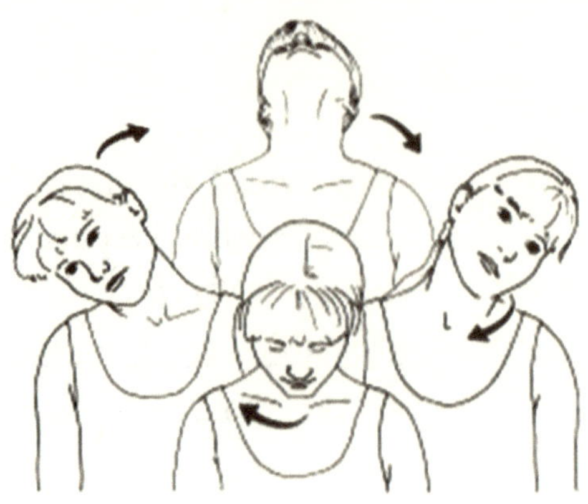

Neck rotate

d) Neck rotation – Rotating the neck half ways clockwise and, anticlockwise.

Neck Strengthening

a) Prone cobra stretch – Lie face down on floor, towel under forehead, pinch shoulder blades together to bring hands off the floor, lift forehead an inch off towel, keep facing down, hold 10 seconds and, back. Repeat five times.

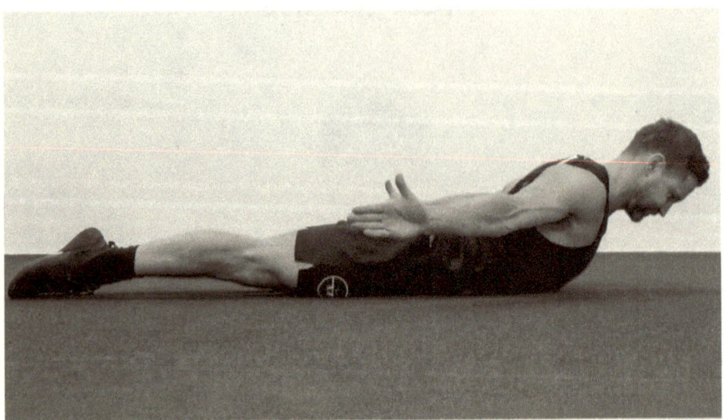

Prone cobra stretch

b) Chin Tuck – Stand with feet shoulder-width apart. Touch your spine to a wall while keeping your head away. Bow your head and, allow it to touch the wall. Hold for 5 seconds. Repeat 10 times.

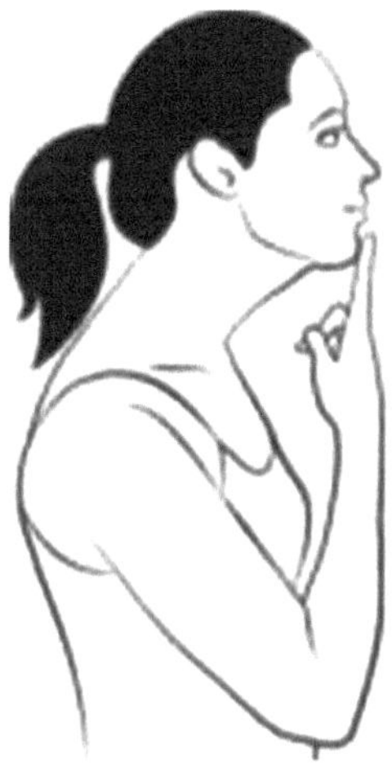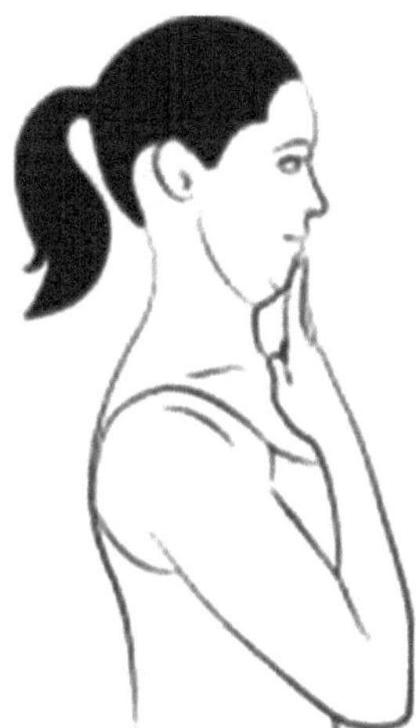

Chin tucks

c) Back Burn- Stand with back against the wall, heels a few inches away. Pull your head back straight and, let it rest against the wall. While still keeping your hands in contact with the wall, bring them up and, over your head and, then back down. Repeat 10 times.

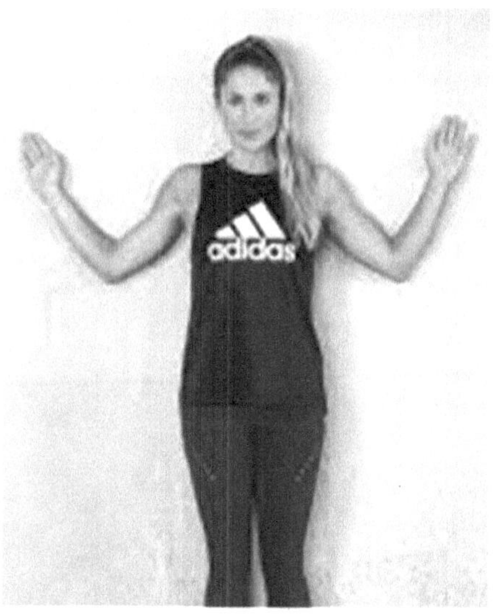

Back burn

Neck pain is common but usually not serious. Your pain should be cured within 2 weeks. Full recovery may take about 4-6 weeks. As your neck starts feeling better, you will be able to resume what you are used to.

There may be other sorts of pain you might suffer from like, ankle, wrist, elbow and, hip joints. Just remember that pain is temporary, don't let it deter you from making progress and, do remember the 7 rules mentioned above.

How to deal with work out related or post work out pain

Suffering from sore muscles a day or two after strenuous exercise or intense work out is very natural, especially if you have just increased the intensity of work out or have started with something new. If you haven't exercised for a while or are starting with a new activity, you are likely to experience sore muscles after work out. This is your body's way of conveying that muscles need time to recover. This pain subsides after 24 to 48 hours of rest. If this doesn't happen, you have either sustained an injury or a muscle sprain.

In case of a sudden injury or pain or sprain after work out first three days you have to put cold pack then if it persist after three days you have to put hot packs. Remember this always.

Tips to relieve muscle pain and, soreness:

❖ Use an ice pack

❖ Go for a massage

❖ Stretch and, cool down properly

❖ Build up exercises slowly

❖ Take a warm bath (A good soak always helps)

CHAPTER 9

SUPPLEMENTS

What are supplements

If any nutrient which can neither be manufactured by our body nor is found in our natural diet, it can be taken as a supplement in prescribed quantities. Food supplements can be vitamins, minerals, carbohydrates, proteins, fatty acids, amino acids and, other substances delivered in form of pills, tablets, capsules, liquids, etc.

Supplements are not a substitute for a balanced healthy diet. A diet that includes plenty of fruits, vegetables, whole grains, adequate protein and, healthy fats should normally provide all the nutrients required for good health.

It has been observed that some people may require supplements because the vitamins and, minerals they need are hard to get in adequate amounts in their diet. This group of people is formed of:

- Pregnant women
- Nursing mother
- Strict vegetarians
- People with food allergies or intolerances
- People of age over 35 years due to their lifestyle
- Certain macros or micros for people having fitness goals

As far as micronutrients, vitamins and, minerals, are concerned; you should definitely get blood tests done and, make the required modifications in your diet as mentioned in the earlier chapters. If this is not possible in your regular diet, take the micronutrients you require in the supplement forms for total health and, better performance in achieving your goals, it's important.

When it comes to macronutrients like proteins, fats and, carbohydrates, it is always preferred to fulfill their requirements through natural diet. But if this is not possible, supplements for these are also available in the markets.

1) ***Whey Protein is a protein supplement***: it is milk protein and, a thus daily product. The whey protein manufacturing undergoes a set of steps as follows –

   a) Milk is derived from cow milk which consists of protein, fat and, lactose.

   b) The unpasteurized milk is cooled at 40 degree Celsius.

   c) Milk is then pasteurized at 72-73 degree Celsius and, then cooled. This is 80% Casein and, 20% whey.

   d) Liquid whey is separated using enzymes. The casein is procured either in the form of various kinds of cheeses or casein protein.

   e) Fat, lactose, minerals and, water are removed from the whey.

   f) This protein is micro filtered to make whey protein concentrate which is further filtered to make whey protein isolate.

   g) This protein is dried to form powder, flavored and, then packed.

If you are not able to fulfill your protein needs from your daily diet, you may take whey protein. Whey protein is generally safe and, can be consumed by almost everyone without side-effects. A commonly suggested dose is 1-2 scoops (around 25-50 grams) per day but it's recommended to follow the serving instruction on the package. Taking more will not offer more benefits especially if you already eat enough protein.

Excessive consumption may lead to digestive issues as some people have lactose intolerance. In that case, you can go for a non-dairy protein powder, such as soy, pea, egg, rice or hemp protein. If you suffer from any kidney related disorders, you must check with your doctor before you begin taking whey protein.

2) ***Fats***: As we have discussed, good fats are really necessary for our health goals. 20% of our diet should have fat in it's unsaturated and, polyunsaturated forms. Please remember that while you need enough veggies, fiber and, other vital nutrients, you also need to include fats in calculated amounts in your diet to achieve your goals.

Two types of polyunsaturated fatty acids are:

Omega 3- flaxseed, canola and, walnut oils, eggs.

Omega 6- found in individually processed oils like, corn and, soybean.

If you feel that your diet is insufficient in fats, these supplements can be taken –

- ❖ Fish oil- Best source of essential omega 3 fatty acids, EPA and, DHA. These fats produce beneficial prostaglandins that inhibit inflammation and, reduce the risk of heart diseases. They also provide other health benefits such as, prevent muscle break down, enhance healing, boost fat loss, enhance muscle count and, improve brain functioning.

- ❖ CLA (Conjugated Linoleic Acid)- It helps to build muscleand strength while simultaneously shedding body fat. It works on the principle of prevention of storage of consumed fat, forcing it to be utilized as fuel. It aids the transport of fat into the mitochondria of the cell, where it is oxidized to obtain energy. This increases the amount of fat burned preventing the muscle from break down which results in greater muscle growth and, strength.

- ❖ GLA (Gama Linolenic acid)- Acts much like Omega 3 as it leads to the production of anti-inflammatory prostaglandins, which have numerous benefits that include better muscle and, joint recovery as well as fat loss.

3) ***Carbohydrates***: Due to many reasons; like time work hours, early morning schedules and, solitary living; cooking becomes an issue and, the carbohydrate needs remain unfulfilled.

In case of carbohydrate deficiency, the body begins to utilize proteins and, fats as a source for energy when the glycogen (stored glucose) reserves get exhausted, which doesn't take much time. Carbohydrates are the body's most preferred source of energy and, you mustn't avoid this group of foods.

In case you are carbohydrate deficient- or suffer from food indigestion-, the following supplements are available in market:

❖ Dextrose- It is essentially pure glucose. It helps in recovering from Zero Digestion. It is sugar in its purest form and, also has a sweet taste.

❖ Maltodextrin- It is actually a polysaccharide that is usually used as a food additive. Though as quick to digest as dextrose, it is not exactly a sugar.

❖ Waxy maize- It is a high molecular weight starch that contains no sugar (sucrose). It is a very unique complex carbohydrate that absorbs very quickly.

These help replenish the glycogen stores of our body.

Carbohydrates - supplemented vs. Natural form

The biggest question at this point is whether you should get your carbohydrates from food or supplements? The answer is a bit surprising. You can get your carbohydrates from both these sources. What actually matters is the time you take them. While supplements can be digested faster than foods, they cause greater insulin spike. Whole foods, on the other hand, will contribute in prevention of recurring hunger spells due to slow digestion. For this very reason, it is better to consume High Glycemic supplement carbohydrates immediately before, during and, after training for better performance. Throughout the day, it is recommended to eat whole foods such as whole grains, fruits and, vegetables.

Performance enhancers which can be added for better results

Performance enhancers help boost your energy and, metabolism and, in turn achieve your fitness goals. These are: Prework out, Fat Burner, Amino Supplement, Test Booster, Glutamine, L- Arginine, L- Carnitine, Multivitamin, Joint Support, Creatine, Vitamin K2, Berberine, Magnesium ZMA, Nitric oxide and, of course, caffeine. All these help in improving our performance and, giving great results.

As mentioned in every list, all the natural sources are present in the supplement list as these are derived from natural sources only and, formulated before being packed for ready to use purposes. But the quantity, expiry and, quality of these products should taken care of.

Let's discuss some of them:

Pre-work out — are multi-ingredient dietary formulas designed to boost energy and, athletic performance. They're typically a powdered substance that you mix in water and, drink before exercise. While countless formulas exist, there's little consistency in terms of ingredients. Amino acids, B vitamins, caffeine, creatine, and, artificial sweeteners are often included, but quantities can vary widely depending on the brand.

Fat Burner - "fat burner" is used to describe "nutrition supplements that are claimed to acutely increase fat metabolism or energy expenditure, impair fat absorption, increase weight loss, increase fat oxidation during exercise, or somehow cause long-term adaptations that promote fat metabolism. Some of the key ingredients used in fat burners are designed to stimulate hormonal reactions in the body, and, to begin breaking down fat and, using it as a fuel source. The main ingredient in most fat burners is caffeine, which helps you lose weight by increasing your metabolism and, helping the body use fat for fuel. It also helps provide energy for exercise and, other calorie-burning activities. In the body, caffeine increases the breakdown of fatty acids that reside in adipose tissue—also known as belly fat. Once the fatty acids are broken down, they enter the bloodstream and, can be burned up by our bodies to create energy.

If you're eating for healthy fat loss, then a thermogenic fat burner can help with the other stuff: boosting energy, helping to curb appetite, promoting fat to be used for energy, and, even increasing your metabolism and, core temperature—what is known as "thermogenesis"—so you burn more calories throughout the day.

Aminos or BCAA - There are 20 different amino acids that make up the thousands of different proteins in the human body. Nine of the 20 are considered essential amino acids, meaning they cannot be made by your body and, must be obtained through your diet. Of the nine essential amino acids, three are the branched-chain amino acids (BCAAs): leucine, isoleucine and, valine. "Branched-chain" refers to the chemical structure of BCAAs, which are found in protein-rich foods such as eggs, meat and, dairy products. They are also a popular dietary supplement sold primarily in powder form.

Test Booster - Testesterone is a hormone that is produced primarily in the testicles for men and, the ovaries and, adrenal glands for women. This hormone is essential to the development of male growth and, masculine characteristics. For women, testosterone comes in much smaller amounts. Testosterone production increases about 30 times more during adolescence and, early adulthood. After early adulthood, it's natural for levels to drop slightly each year. Your body may see a one percent decline after you're 30 years old.

Testosterone plays a key role in your:

❖ muscle mass and, bones

❖ facial and, pubic hair

❖ body's development of deeper voices

❖ sex drive

❖ mood and, quality of life

❖ verbal memory and, thinking ability

L Carnitine - L-carnitine can boost both your training and, your physique. In the gym, it can mean more endurance and, bigger pumps. In the mirror, picture more muscle and, less fat. While it is often categorized as an amino acid, L-carnitine isn't technically an amino. It is considered a "vitamin-like" and, "amino-acid-like" compound that is related to the B vitamins. When it was first studied back in the 1950s, L-carnitine was referred to as vitamin BT.

L-carnitine is formed in the liver and, kidneys from the amino acids lysine and, methionine. However, it is stored elsewhere in the body, primarily in muscle (including the heart), the brain, and, even in sperm. In the diet, it mainly comes from meat and, other animal products. You can get some from plant products like avocado and, soybeans, but as a rule, meat is the best source—and, the redder the better.

Glutamine - Glutamine is the most common amino acid found in your muscles—over 61% of skeletal muscle is Glutamine. Glutamine consists of 19% nitrogen, making it the primary transporter of nitrogen into your muscle cells.

During intense training, Glutamine levels are greatly depleted in your body, which decreases strength, stamina and, recovery. It could take up to 6 days for Glutamine levels to return to normal—and, Glutamine plays a key role in protein synthesis. Studies have shown that L-Glutamine supplementation can minimize breakdown of muscle and, improve protein metabolism.

L Arginine - L-arginine is one of many amino acids the body needs to function properly. Like other amino acids, L-arginine plays a role in building protein. The body can use the protein to help build muscle and, rebuild tissue.

As a result, researchers have investigated the effectiveness of L-arginine in the treatment of severe wounds and, tissue waste in serious illnesses.

Multi Vitamin - Multivitamins are a combination of many different **vitamins** that are normally found in foods and, other natural sources. Multivitamins are used to provide **vitamins** that are not taken in through the diet. Multivitamins are also used to treat vitamin deficiencies (lack of **vitamins**) caused by illness, pregnancy, poor nutrition, digestive disorders, and, many other conditions.

Joint Support – Many people deal with chronic joint pain in their knees, hands, elbows, shoulders, and, elsewhere. In most cases, this is caused by the most common type of arthritis, osteoarthritis. This form of arthritis affects almost entire population. Pain relievers such as acetaminophen (Tylenol) or nonsteroidal anti-inflammatory drugs, such as ibuprofen (Advil), are usually the first choice for joint pain relief. here are also dozens of supplements that claim to treat joint pain, but which ones actually work

Some of them are – calcium, glucosamine, chrondroitin,

ZMA - ZMA, or zinc magnesium aspartate, is a popular supplement among athletes, bodybuilders, and, fitness enthusiasts. It contains a combination of three ingredients — zinc, magnesium, and, vitamin B6. ZMA manufacturers claim it boosts muscle growth and, strength and, improves endurance, recovery, and, sleep quality.

Fish oil - Omega-3 fish oil contains both docosahexaenoic acid (DHA) and, eicosapentaenoic acid (EPA). Omega-3 fatty acids are essential nutrients that are important in preventing and, managing heart disease.

Findings show omega-3 fatty acids may help to:

- ❖ Lower blood pressure
- ❖ Reduce triglycerides
- ❖ Slow the development of plaque in the arteries
- ❖ Reduce the chance of abnormal heart rhythm
- ❖ Reduce the likelihood of heart attack and, stroke
- ❖ Lessen the chance of sudden cardiac death in people with heart disease

These performance enhancers can be used with proper guidance, and, they will definitely help in achieving your targets.

CHAPTER 10

MIND IS THE MOST IMPORTANT TOOL

Mind Is The Most Important Tool

"A well built physique is more than vanity. It shows discipline, dignity and, dedication. It requires patience, passion and, self-respect. It cannot be bought, stolen or inherited. It cannot be held without constant work."

– M. Arnold Schwarzenegger

"Strength does not come from winning. Your struggles develop your strengths. When you go through hardships and, still decide not to surrender, that is strength."

– M. Arnold Schwarzenegger

In my fitness career, I came across many people that were unable to continue with this regime and, their dream of a good physique remained just that, a dream. It's not that they were incapable of doing it, they just left things in between. It's just like drawing a picture or going on a journey.

When you decide to create a picture, you do the following;

1) Firstly, you select an image, one that you either envision or see. It can be a good scenery, a celebrity sketch, a monument or anything that you feel you can bring out on a sheet of paper beautifully.

2) Then, you collect the required materials for accomplishing the task. Pencils, canvas or a simple sheet of paper, colours etc. and, find you a good place to sit down and, work.

3) The guidelines or knowledge required for completing your picture is with you before you begin.

4) Time. If you do not draw or paint for a living, you'll have to take out time for the task every day.

5) Every day is not the same; you need motivation and, inspiration to continue painting.

6) At times, you run out of the required material or motivation. You simply cannot continue and, so draw something less concrete that you know you will erase and, make again someday.

7) Having been consistent and, informed, one day you will finally finish that picture and, smile to yourself. It is finally done and, you find that you are very happy.

Your fitness goals are similar to drawing a picture.

Like creating a picture, you have to create a new you. You need to invest time efforts and, money with consistency, commitment, dedication and, hard work, that too daily, 24 hours x 365 days in a year.

Yes, that's how it is done.

Its not about just going to a gym, a park or an aerobic class or a yoga studio for just an hour and, forget it. Body transformation is a 24 hour thing, every second of the day matters. Your work out, meals, sleep, daily activities, rest, everything matters. Daily progression is the key.

Today you did 3 km in 25 minutes, tomorrow or in next schedule you have to either reduce the time or increase the distance. Today you did 12 repetitions with 10kg, tomorrow or next schedule 14 reps with the same weight. Today you stretched to one point, in next session you have to push further. It is this way.

Same is the case in your meals. You have to calculate each and, every calorie you eat, or I would say each and, every meal is pre calculated, it is scheduled and, fixed.

I know this is tough, but if you want to fulfill your dreams, it is important. Let me tell you it is not a five year project, more you are flexible with your routines, more it will be tough, challenging and, time consuming. Just give your best once, may be six months or a year depending on your targets, and, then you can easily maintain it.

Its all in mind. You have to convince yourself first and, then you will be able to convince people around you.

Social pressure or the family pressure is the biggest enemy I have seen, because of which people leave their journey in between. Let me tell you one thing, you are working on something, because you feel its important for you, why will any body else feel it's important. Their priorities are different from you and, they are working on them. It's your journey and, you have to complete it. What ever it takes, you have to give.

There will be people around you who will stop you or give their comments on daily basis. But you don't have to listen. You either have to convince them or you have to be blunt in saying that, it's my journey. Fitness demands consistency. Daily you have to take out time for your work outs, meals, you have to either avoid parties or you have to eat in your own way at the get together and, functions.

There will be a lot of criticism, at times humiliations also, but you have to ignore it and, move on.

In work outs, we always say everyday is not Monday, yes you would not have the same energy levels daily. You have to fulfill other duties also and, a daily routine is to be followed too. At times it will be late nights, at times meals will also not be popular. It is ok, it happens, but in any case you have to balance your work outs and, your daily life.

Physical discomfort is an integral part of this body transformation journey. Strenuous work outs and, calculated meals, will definitely make you tired and, sore. But You have to move on towards your goals. At times you have to deal with body pain, when you will not be able to work out also, trust me its ok, its part of the journey. It had been many times that throughout the journey you have to take rest for certain days and, at times for months also, I have done it many times, but in that case it should be active rest. The diet will still be calculated, and, keeping in mind all the calculations you to move ahead. I really remember once when I was preparing for a competition, I injured myself badly and, that too twice in a month, but I never stopped my work out, I altered my schedule, I would go to the gym, and, do what all I was able to. Here I will mention that when my knee got injured I was not able to do endurance training, in that case I used to do super sets for the upper body so that I could sweat to the maximum.

Many a times I have seen people that they get disturbed from small things, like a day off, a cheat meal or a missed meal, a bad work out. It is really fine. It all happens. You can always cover up.

Trust me your body is capable to achieve anything, its just your mind you need to convince.

In the end, Here I am giving six rules of body transformation which I followed throughout my life and, they will help you to succeed no matter what the circumstances are –

1. ***Fitness should the your priority*** – No matter what I do, fitness is my first priority. I have never said to myself, I want to sleep so I can't go for a cardio session or I have to make others happy, so I can not maintain my diet or he or she is not happy with my training routines so I will not be able to continue. No, It's my priority, I will do it.

2. ***Motivation is the key*** – I never felt de motivated, no matter how much time it takes, no matter what people say, no matter how dissatisfying the results were. I was always positive about my fitness regime and, my goals.

3. ***Never listen U Can't*** – I only listen to people and, words which encouraged me to move further, and, never ever heard to people who said "you can't do it"

4. ***Work out as if there's no tomorrow*** – After my every work out I was actually not able to breathe or I would vomit, just gave my best in every work out session and, tried to perform better than the previous day.

5. ***Stomach is not a dustbin*** – 99.99%, I never ate, something which doesn't favor my fitness goals, not in my daily life and, not even in get-togethers or parties. I could really remember many parties where I was sitting with a glass of water for hours.

6. ***Protect your dream*** – My dream is like my kid, I protected it from the entire world. My kid cried many a times, but I was there for him always, and, the dream became a reality.

My idol Mr. Arnold Schwazzeneger says,

"If I can see it and, believe it, then I can ACHIEVE IT"

CHAPTER 11

SAMPLE WORK OUT PLANS FOR ALL BODY TYPES

Here I would like to mention that the schedules mentioned for all the body types are for beginner to intermediate to advance levels, depending on the capacity of the person and, how much time you have been doing work outs.

One thing need to be taken care by people who have just started with their work outs, you have to start with 50% of the volume mentioned in the schedules and, gradually as you get stamina and, strength you can increase the volume of the training.

Like in endurance training, if it is written 40 minutes, start with 20 minutes and, gradually increase it.

In strength if its written 3 sets or 2 sets, begin with one set and, try doing all the exercises, rather then emphasizing on one exercise.

In flexibility training stretch your self within comfort zone and, gradually increase the intensity.

Learn to have patience when it comes to be adaptive, you have been less active in the previous days, your body needs time to get used to it with new work outs.

Remember you have to get fit, then only you will be able to look fit.

Sample work out plans for all body types

Sample Work out Schedule for Category 1 – Ectomorph – Without any equipment – Five days a week

Day 1

Warm Up and, Stretching

Neck Rotation – 10 clock wise and, 10 anticlockwise

Shoulder rotation 10 forward and, 10 backward

Shoulder, bicep, triceps, chest, back stretches as mentioned

Forward Bending and, standing back stretch – 5 times

Spine twist – 5 each side

Standing front thigh stretch

Standing Gluteus stretch

Now work out starts

1. Pushups 10 x 5 sets
2. Squats 20 x 5 sets
3. Pull ups – As many repetitions as possible (AMRAP)
4. Planks – 1miniute x 3 sets

    Cool down – repeat the warm up routine

Day 2

20 to 40 minutes steady state endurance training (fast walking, running, cycling, stair climbing or any other any kind of sports activity done in continuous manner)

Day 3

11 Suryanamaskar

Day 4

Warm up and, stretch

Super Set the following

Burpees 10 reps

Sumo squats 20 reps

Diamond Pushups 10 reps

Total 3 rounds of the above combination

Super Set the following

Parallel lunges 10 each side

Mount climb 15 each side

Inverted Rows or table pull ups – 10

Total 3 rounds of the above combination

Cycling crunches 20 each sides x 3 sets

Hyper extension – 10 reps x 3 sets

Cool down and, stretch

Day 5

Flexibilty training

Hold each stretch for 1 minutes and, repeat 3 to 5 times

1. Sit and, Reach
2. Toe Touch.
3. Groin stretch
4. Lateral side Bending
5. Trunk Rotation stretch
6. Shoulder Stretch
7. Hip Rotators stretch

2 sets suryanamaskar

The above mentioned schedule is a sample schedule

Repititions and, sets can be increased gradually with time as the strength increases

Similar exercises can be chosen from the exercises mentioned in the exercise section in previous chapters.

Sample Work out Schedule for Category 1 – Ectomorph – With equipment(dumbbell, barbell, weights or strength rope) – Five days a week

Warm up, Stretch and, cool down Daily as mentioned above and, in flexibility routines

Day 1

After warm up

Pushups – 10 reps x 3 sets

Barbell Bench Press – repetitions 12,8,8,6

Front shoulder barbell Press – reps – 12,8,8

Standing side laterals for shoulders – 8 x 3 sets

Pullovers 12 x 3 sets

Overhead dumbbell triceps extensions – 8 x 3 sets

Triceps Pulley push downs

Crunches 20 x 3 sets

Leg raises – 20 x 3 sets

Hyper extensions 10 x 3 sets

Day 2

20 to 40 minutes steady state endurance training (fast walking, running, cycling, stair climbing or any other any kind of sports activity done in continuous manner)

Day 3

Wide Grip chin-ups – 30 to 50 reps in sets

Upright Rowing with barbell – 12,8,8

Seated Rowing – 8,8,8

One arm dumbbell rows – 8,8,8

Good Mornings – 10x3 sets

Standing Barbell biceps curls – 16,12,8,8

Inclined alternate dumbbell bicep curls – 8,8,6

Cycling Crunches 50 reps each side

Day 4

30 minutes endurance training and, 30 minutes flexibility routine as mentioned above

Day 5

4 sets suryanamaskar

50 free squats

Weighted squats – 20,16,12,8,8

Dead lift -20,16,12,12

Static lunges – 10 each side x 3 sets

Leg extensions 10 x 3 sets

Leg curls 20,16,12

1 set suryanamaskar.

Sample Work out Schedule for Category 2 – Ecto Meso morph – Without any equipment – Five days a week

Day 1

20 to 40 minutes steady state endurance training (fast walking, running, cycling, stair climbing or any other any kind of sports activity done in continuous manner) followed by flexibility training for 10 to 20 minutes

Day 2

Warm Up and, Stretching

Neck Rotation – 10 clock wise and, 10 anticlockwise

Shoulder rotation 10 forward and, 10 backward

Shoulder, bicep, triceps, chest, back stretches as mentioned

Forward Bending and, standing back stretch – 5 times

Spine twist – 5 each side

Standing front thigh stretch

Standing Gluteus stretch

Now work out starts

Combo 1 – all three exercises in circuit 4 times

Pushups – 10 reps x 4 sets

Superset with

Squats – 15 reps x 4 sets

Super set with

sit ups level 1 or 2 as comfortable – 10 reps x 4 sets

Combo 2 – all three exercise in circuit 4 times

Dips behind the back 10 reps x 4 sets

Superset with

Reverse lunges with knee lifts – 10 reps each side x 4 sets

Superset with

Plank – 1minutes x 4 sets

Cool down and, repeat the warm up routine

Day 3

20 to 40 minutes steady state endurance training (fast walking, running, cycling, stair climbing or any other any kind of sports activity done in continuous manner) followed by flexibility training for 10 to 20 minutes

Day 4

Warm up and, stretch as mentioned

Combo 1- all three exercise 4 times

Wide grip pushups – 15 reps x 4 sets

Mount climb – 15 each side x 4 sets

Gluteus Bridge single leg – 15 each side x 4 sets

Combo 2 – All three exercises in a series 4 times

Table pull ups 10 reps x 4 sets

Wide or sumo squats – 20 x 4 sets

Single leg dead lift – 15 each side x 4 sets

Cool down and, stretch

Day 5

30 minute Endurance training and, after that 11 suryanamaskar with 4 mount climb in every suryanamaskar.

Sample Work out Schedule for Category 2 – Ecto Meso morph – With equipments – Five days a week

Day1, Day3, Day 5

Will be same as above mentioned in ectomesomorph category

Day2

Warm up and, stretching as mentioned above

Barbell Bench chest press – 16,12,8,8

Inclines Bench Barbell press 16,12,12

Front Shoulder Dumbbell press 12 x 3 sets

Standing Barbell Bicep Curls 12,8,8

Front shoulder raises 12,8,8

Leg extensions 8x3 sets

Lunges – 10 each side x 3 sets

Cycling crunches – 20 each side x 3 sets

Reverse crunches 30 x 3 sets

Cool down and, stretching

Day 4

Warm up and, stretching as mentioned

Good morning 10 x 3 sets

Squats 20,16,12,12

Dead lift – 20, 16 12 12

Wide Grip pull ups - Total 50 reps in minimum breaks or sets or Lat pull downs – 16,12,12,8

Close grip pull ups – 30 reps in minimum sets superset with pull overs 15 x 3 sets

Seated Rowing – 16,12,8

Upright rowing 12,8,8

Shoulder side laterals – 10 x 3 sets

Standing or seated overhead triceps barbell or dumbbell extensions 8 x 3 sets

Leg Raises – 50 reps

Cool down and, stretch

Sample Work out Schedule for Category 3 – Meso morph – Without equipments – Five days a week

Warm up and, stretch your full body daily as mentioned in above categories

Day 1

20 to 40 minutes steady state endurance training (fast walking, running, cycling, stair climbing or any other any kind of sports activity done in continuous manner)

The following four exercises in a circuit – total 3 to 5 rounds

Mount Climb – 30 each side

Alternate leg raises - 20 each side

Walking lunges – 10 each side

Pushups – 10 to 20 reps

Cool down and, stretch

Day 2

Suryanamaskar – start with 5 reps each side than increase it to 11 reps

The following four exercises in a circuit – total 3 to 5 rounds

Elbow plank to full plank shift – 10 reps each side

Russian twist on floor – 20 each side

Parallel lunges side to side – 10 each side

Cool down and, stretch

Day 3

40 to 60 minutes steady state endurance training (fast walking, running, cycling, stair climbing or any other any kind of sports activity done in continuous manner)

Day 4

The following five exercises in a circuit – total 3 to 5 rounds

Jumping Jacks – 30 reps

Burpees – 20 reps

Side dribble with toe touch 10 each side

On the spot high knee run – 50 counts

Single leg glute bridge – 30 seconds hold

Now the following exercises

Plank – 1 minutes x 5 sets

Oblique crunches – 30 counts x 3 sets

Hyper extensions – 20 reps x 3 sets

Cool down

Day 5

40 to 60 minutes steady state endurance training (fast walking, running, cycling, stair climbing or any other any kind of sports activity done in continuous manner)

Sample Work out Schedule for Category 3 – Meso morph – With equipments – Five days a week

Day 1 and, 2 will be same as above mentioned in without equipment section

Day 3

Wide grip Chin ups – 30 to 50 reps

Close grip chin-ups – 30 reps

Pullovers – 20 reps x 3sets

Seated rowing – 20,16,12

One arm dumbbell rowing – 20,16,12

Upright rowing – 16,12,8

Rear deltoid laterals – 20,16,16

Dead lift – 20,16,12,8

Hanging leg rises – 20 reps x 5 sets

Sit ups – 10 x 5 sets

Seated twists – 50 reach side

30 minutes endurance training steady state, any form, cycling, jogging etc

Day 4

2 sets Suryanamaskar

Free Squats – 50reps

Weighted barbell or dumbbell press or leg press – 25,20,16,12

Leg extensions 10 x 3 sets

Leg curls – 20,16,16,12

Lunges static – 10 reps each side x 4 sets

Sumo squats with dumbbell – 12 x 3 sets

Hyper extensions on floor – 20 x 3 sets

20 minutes endurance training

Weighted Calf raises – 10 reps x 3 sets

Cool down

Day 5

Flat bench Barbell press – 20,16,12,12

Inclined bench barbell press – 20, 16, 12, 12

Flat chest fly – 12 x 3 sets

Bar dips – 15 x 3 sets

Front barbell shoulder press – 12 x 3 sets

Front raises – 12 x 3 sets

Shoulder dumbbell side laterals – 12 x 3 sets

Compound crunches – 30 x 3 sets

Plank twist – 20 each side x 3 sets

Good mornings 10 reps x 3 sets

Sample Work out Schedule for Category 4 – Meso Endomorph – Without equipments – Five days a week

Warm up and, stretch your full body daily as mentioned in above categories

Day 1

40 to 60 minutes steady state endurance training (fast walking, running, cycling, stair climbing or any other any kind of sports activity done in continuous manner)

The following four exercises in a circuit – total 3 to 5 rounds

Mount Climb – 30 each side

Alternate leg raises - 20 each side

Walking lunges – 10 each side

Pushups – 10 to 20 reps

Cool down and, stretch

Day 2

Suryanamaskar – start with 5 reps each side than increase it to 11 reps

The following four exercises in a circuit – total 3 to 5 rounds

Elbow plank to full plank shift – 10 reps each side

Russian twist on floor – 20 each side

Parallel lunges side to side – 10 each side

Cool down and, stretch

Day 3

40 to 60 minutes steady state endurance training (fast walking, running, cycling, stair climbing or any other any kind of sports activity done in continuous manner)

Day 4

The following five exercises in a circuit – total 3 to 5 rounds

Jumping Jacks – 30 reps

Burpees – 20 reps

Side dribble with toe touch 10 each side

On the spot high knee run – 50 counts

Single leg glute bridge – 30 seconds hold

Now the following exercises

Plank – 1 minutes x 5 sets

Oblique crunches – 30 counts x 3 sets

Hyper extensions – 20 reps x 3 sets

Cool down

Day 5

40 to 60 minutes steady state endurance training (fast walking, running, cycling, stair climbing or any other any kind of sports activity done in continuous manner)

Sample Work out Schedule for Category 4 – Meso Endo morph – With equipments – Six days a week

Day 1

20 MINUTES Endurance training

INCLINED CRUNCHES 15 x 3 sets

MOUNT CLIMB 20 each side x 3 sets

TWISTED LEG LIFTS – 10 each side x 3 sets

STRETCH FOR 2 MINUTES

DIVEBOMB PUSHUPS – 25 X 2 SETS

FLAT BENCH BARBELL PRESS – 25,20,15

INCLINED BENCH BARBELL PRESS – 25,20, 15

FLAT DUMBELL PRESS WITH DUMBELL ROTATION – 15 X 3 SETS

PULLOVERS – 20 X 3 SETS

LYING BARBELL TRICEP EXTENSIONS WITH CLOSE GRIP PUSHUPS – 20,20,16,16

COOL DOWN AND, STRETCH

DAY 2

3 KM RUN ON TREADMILL IN MINUMUM TIME

ALL THREE BELOW MENTIONED EXERCISES IN SERIES (TOTAL 4 ROUNDS)

200 INCLINED BOARD REVERSE CRUNCHES WITH HIP LIFT (50 X 4 SETS)

100 EACH SIDE KNEE ELBOW TOUCH AND, KICK UPWARDS (25 X 4 SETS)

HALF PLANK JACKS – 100 EACH SIDE (25 X 4 SETS)

NOW THE FOLLOWING WORK OUT

LAT MACHINE PULL DOWN BEHIND THE NECK – 25,20,16,16

DEADLIFT – 30,25,20,16

BENT OVER DUMBELL ROWS – 20,20,16,16

FACEPULLS – 20 X 3 SETS

GOOD MORNINGS – 10X3 SETS

CROSS FACE TRICEP EXTENSIONS – 12,8,8,4

COOL DOWN AND, STRETCH

DAY 3

CROSSTRAINER – 45 MINUTES

TREADMILL – 20 MINUTES

BICYCLE CRUNCHES – 100 REPS IN ONE GO

BURPEES – 50 IN ONE GO

100 SQUATS IN ONE GO

2 SETS SURYANAMASKAR

COOL DOWN

DAY 4

LOWER BODY STRETCHING

LEG CURLS – 30,20,16,12,12 + STIFF LEG DEADLIFT – 30,25,20,16,16

SQUATS – 30,25,20,20

LEG EXTENSIONS – 20 X 4 SETS

SIDE LUNGES – 50 COUNTS

SIDE LEG RAISES WITH WEIGHTS – 20X3 SETS

ONE LEGGED DUMBELL ROWING – 10X 3 SETS EACH SIDE

SINGLE DUMBELL DEADLIFT – 10X3 SETS

WEIGHTED CALF RAISES – 10 X 3 SETS (WEIGHT EQUAL TO BODYWEIGHT)

2 SETS SURYANAMASKAR AND, 10 MINUTES COOL DOWN

DAY 5

CROSSTRAINER – 45 MINUTES

TREADMILL – 20 MINUTES

BICYCLE CRUNCHES – 100 REPS IN ONE GO

BURPEES – 50 IN ONE GO

100 SQUATS IN ONE GO

2 SETS SURYANAMASKAR

DAY 6

WARM UP AND, STRETCHING

3KM TREADMILL

ALL BELOWMENTIONED THREE EXERCISES IN A ROW – TOTAL 4 ROUNDS

LEG WIPERS 25 X 4 SETS

SINGLE LEG GLUTE BRIDGES LIFT – 25 EACH SIDE X 4 SETS

NAUKA ASAN – 1MIN HOLD X 4 SETS

SWIMMERS – 20 X 4 SETS

BODY PARTS TO TRAIN – SHOULDERS AND, BICEPS

ARNOLD PRESSES - - 8X3 SETS

BEHIND THE NECK BARBELL PRESSES – 12,8,8

CLEAN AND, PRESS – 6,6,4

ONE ARM CROSS CABLE LATERALS – 8X3 SETS

REVERSE OVERHEAD DUMBELL LATERALS

PREACHER CURLS WITH DUMBELL – 12,8,8,6

INCLINE DUMBELL 3 PART CURLS (21S) – 4 SETS

COOL DOWN AND, STRETCH

Sample Work out Schedule for Category 5 – Endomorph – Without equipments – Five days a week

Warm up and, stretch your full body daily as mentioned in above categories

Day 1

40 to 60 minutes steady state endurance training (fast walking, running, cycling, stair climbing or any other any kind of sports activity done in continuous manner)

The following four exercises in a circuit – total 3 to 5 rounds

Planks – 30 seconds to 1 min

Pushups – 10 to 20 reps

Squats – 20 reps

Cool down and, stretch

Day 2

Suryanamaskar – start with 5 reps each side than increase it to 11 reps

20 minutes endurance training

Cool down and, stretch

Day 3

40 to 60 minutes steady state endurance training (fast walking, running, cycling, stair climbing or any other any kind of sports activity done in continuous manner)

Day 4

The following five exercises in a circuit – total 3 to 5 rounds

Half Jumping Jacks – 30 reps

Half Burpees – 20 reps

Side dribble with toe touch 10 each side

On the spot high knee run – 50 counts

Single leg glute bridge – 30 seconds hold

Now the following exercises

Plank – 1 minutes x 5 sets

Oblique crunches – 30 counts x 3 sets

Hyper extensions – 20 reps x 3 sets

Cool down

Day 5

40 to 60 minutes steady state endurance training (fast walking, running, cycling, stair climbing or any other any kind of sports activity done in continuous manner)

Sample Work out Schedule for Category 5 – Endo morph – With equipments – five days a week

Day 1

Warm up 2 km in minimum time

Cross fit work out

Plank knee elbow 15 each side + full crunches on incline board with plate 20reps + seated tucks on floor with dumbbell spacing 30 reps - **Total 4 rounds of this combo**

- ❖ Lying Leg Curls   2 Sets 30 Reps
- ❖ Stiif Leg Dumbbell Deadlift

- ❖ c/w Elevated Leg Hip Thrust   2 Sets 30 Reps
- ❖ Barbell Squat c/w Leg Extension   2 Sets 30 Reps
- ❖ Hack Squat c/w Leg Press   2 Sets 30 Reps
- ❖ Split leg good mornings 2 sets 15 rep each side
- ❖ Calf Raises on Leg Press   2 Sets 20 Reps
- ❖ Standing dumbell curls with lying tricep ext 4 sets 30 reps
- ❖ Inclined dumbbell curls with one arm tricep ext 4 sets 20 reps each

40 minute endurance training

Day 2

Warm up and, stretch

Mount climb 50 each side +burpee 20 counts +side dribble with 2 jumping jacks 10 reps +high knee up

Total 4 rounds of the above circuit

- ❖ Pushups s/w Inverted Rows   2 Sets   Max Reps
- ❖ Inclined Dumbbell Press s/w
- ❖ Bent Over Dumbbell Rows   2 Sets   30 Reps
- ❖ Machine Press s/w Seated Rows   2 Sets   30 Reps
- ❖ Flat Dumbbell Fly s/w Bent Over Lateral Raise   2 Sets   30 Reps
- ❖ Lat Pulldown s/w Front Barbell Press   2 Sets   30 Reps
- ❖ Dumbbell Lateral Raise s/w
- ❖ Dumbbell Front Raise   2 Sets   30 Reps
- ❖ Upright Rows   3 Sets   30 Reps

20 minutes endurance training

Day 3

40 to 60 minutes endurance training

21 suryanamaskar

Seated twist 100 each side

Leg raises – 30 counts x 4 sets

Leg wipers – 20 each sides x 4 sets

Cool down

Day 4

Warm up and, Stretch

- ❖ Planks 90 secs s/w close grip pull downs 30, 25 2 Sets
- ❖ Flat dumbell Press

s/w Barbell Back Shoulder Press

s/w Bent Over Barbell Rows

s/w Barbell Curls

s/w Triceps Overhead Dumbbell Extension 2 Sets 30 Reps each Exercise

- ❖ Inclined Dumbbell Fly

s/w Chest Supported Dumbbell Swings

s/w Lat Pulldown

s/w Hammer Curls

s/w Triceps Pushdown 2 Sets 30 Reps each Exercise

- ❖ CYCLING HIGH-INTENSITY 20 Minutes

Day 5

Warm up 2 km in minimum time

Cross fit work out

Plank knee elbow 15 each side + full crunches on incline board with plate 20reps + seated tucks on floor with dumbbell spacing 30 reps - Total 4 rounds of this combo

Now 4 rounds of the below mentioned combo

Plank knee elbow 15 each side + full crunches on incline board with plate 20reps + seated tucks on floor with dumbbell spacing 30 reps

30 minutes endurance training